UNSAFE AT ANY MEAL

What the FDA Does Not Want You
To Know About the Foods You Eat

UNSAFE AT ANY MEAL

What the FDA Does Not Want You
To Know About the Foods You Eat

DR. RENEE JOY DUFAULT

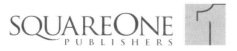
SQUAREONE
PUBLISHERS

The information and advice contained in this book are based upon the research and the personal and professional experiences of the author. They are not intended as a substitute for consulting with a health care professional. The publisher and author are not responsible for any adverse effects or consequences resulting from the use of any of the suggestions, preparations, or procedures discussed in this book. All matters pertaining to your physical health should be supervised by a health care professional. It is a sign of wisdom, not cowardice, to seek a second or third opinion.

COVER DESIGNER: Jeannie Tudor
EDITOR: Caroline Smith
TYPESETTER: Gary A. Rosenberg

Square One Publishers

115 Herricks Road
Garden City Park, NY 11040
(516) 535-2010 • (877) 900-BOOK • www.squareonepublishers.com

Library of Congress Cataloging-in-Publication Data

Names: Dufault, Renee, author.
Title: Unsafe at any meal : what consumers must know to protect their families /
    by Renee Dufault.
Description: Garden City Park, NY : Square One Publishers, 2017. |
    Includes bibliographical references and index.
Identifiers: LCCN 2017000561 (print) | LCCN 2017007917 (ebook) |
    ISBN 9780757004360 (pbk. : alk. paper) | ISBN 9780757054365
Subjects: LCSH: Nutrition. | Food—Toxicology. | Food—Safety measures. |
    Consumer education.
Classification: LCC RA784 .D84 2017 (print) | LCC RA784 (ebook) |
    DDC 613.2—dc23
LC record available at https://lccn.loc.gov/2017000561

ISBN: 978-0-7570-0436-0 (pb)
ISBN: 978-0-7570-5436-5 (eBook)

Printed in the United States of America

10   9   8   7   6   5   4   3   2   1

Contents

*For my children, grandchildren,
and the next generation.*

Acknowledgments

This book is a long time coming but not overdue. The state of research is now at a point where I could write it with confidence. Many individuals have contributed to the mercury research, either directly or indirectly, or helped to disseminate the results in one way or another through the years. I would like to thank all of the following individuals for doing their part:

Blaise LeBlanc, Ed Rau, Boyd Haley, Sree Kumar, Chuck Cornett, Alex and Lyudmila Romanyukha, Chad Mitchell, Bill Walsh, Walter Lukiw, Matt Amann, Don Demers, Martha Boss, Dennis Day, Art Dungan, Isaac Pessah, Peter Green, David Krabbenhoft, Cynthia Harris, Barry Lai, Roseanne Schnoll, Laura Schweitzer, David Wallinga, Fred and Alice Ottoboni, Jane Hightower, Lyn Patrick, Rao Ivaturi, Steven Gilbert, Raquel Crider, Leah Woodke, Amanda Hitt, Melinda Wenner, Scott Laster, Martha Herbert, Katsi Cook, David Carpenter, Matt Pamuku, Skip Kingston, Marcia Zimmerman, Daniele Pisanello, Ted Levine, David and Jamie Fletcher, Tom Devine, The Buss Family, Ivan Royster, Mari Eggers, Maureen Swanson, Marissa McInnis, Zara Berg, Erica Newland, Twila Martin-Kekahbah, Larry Wetsit, Wayne Two Bulls, Mesay Mulugeta Wolle, GM Mizanur Rahman, Alika Maunakea, Dan Laks, and the Fort Peck Community College (FPCC) students who participated in the recent clinical trial that focused on the prevention of type 2 diabetes through the elimination of toxic substances from the diet and increased intake of whole, healthy foods.

Thank you also to my editor, Caroline Smith, a talented writer, who helped me organize the contents of the book to make it easier for the public to read, and Rudy Shur, my publisher and friend, who believed in me from the very start and is committed to helping me get this information out to the public.

Foreword

We understand both more and less about the impact of what we eat on our health and well-being. There are several problems that cloud our vision and inhibit useful action. First, there has never been adequate research on understanding our basic nutritional needs. Furthermore, national nutritional guidelines are affected by food industry and political consideration.

Second, the farm government subsidy program influences the prices of the food we eat. For example, subsiding grain and corn makes the production of beef less expensive and sweetened beverages cheaper.

Third, the mass production and distribution of food results in the use of more chemicals such as pesticides, preservatives, and other additives, that contaminate our food supply. The health effects of some of these chemicals have been studied, but in most cases we lack basic research on the effects of these chemicals from conception through adulthood and aging.

Fourth, we have become increasingly aware that kids are not little adults and that their developing organ systems are more vulnerable to industrial chemicals. In addition, kids eat more, breathe more, and drink more per body weight than adults, which mean they are both exposed to more chemicals and receive a greater dose than adults.

Fifth, there is a complex regulatory structure that attempts to ensure the safety and adequacy of the food supply but suffers from lack of funding while being buffeted by the competing interests of consumers, industry, and politics.

Finally, the greatest challenge is empowering consumers with adequate knowledge and motivation to make choices that protect and promote the health and well-being of not only their families, but also the greater environment. Even more salient is how to protect our children and ensure they have access to food that allows them to reach and maintain their full potential.

The essence of Renee Dufault's book *Unsafe at Any Meal* is captured in the subtitle "What Consumers Must Know to Protect Their Families." An admirable element of this book is that it is grounded in science and extensively referenced. If you want more details or background information, the references listed in the back of the book provide a starting point. This book does a fantastic job of connecting the dots between the science and everyday actions that can be taken to apply what you have learned. I hope every reader takes this information to heart and follows the guidelines in Chapter 8. The relentless focus on what we are eating and what's in what we are eating is essential to making changes in our diet and improving our health. Clearly after reading this book, the conclusion has to be that the underlying science is complicated. However, Renee provides essential guidance and offers simple ways to alter your diet to reduce chemical and heavy metal exposures that will most certainly improve your and your family's health. I hope after reading this book and examining your diet that you have started on a journey that will lead to better health and a more sustainable environment.

Dr. Steven G. Gilbert, Ph.D., DABT, *is a leading researcher in the field of toxicology. He is the director and founder of the Institute of Neurotoxicology and Neurological Disorders based in Seattle, Washington. Dr. Gilbert serves as a director on a number of non-profit organization boards to include among others the Food Ingredient and Health Research Institute and Physicians for Social Responsibility.*

Preface

It took nearly ten years, but a connection has finally been made between eating processed food and inorganic mercury exposure. A team of researchers and I analyzed thirteen years of data and conducted a clinical trial in which human subjects reduced their intake of processed foods. We found they had lower inorganic blood mercury levels compared with subjects who did not significantly reduce their processed food intake.[1] In other words, we simply demonstrated that eating processed foods contributes to higher inorganic blood mercury levels.[1] This means the more processed food you eat, the higher your inorganic blood mercury levels will be.

Why should you care? Inorganic mercury exposure can make you more prone to disease—for example, inorganic mercury exposure increases your risk of type 2 diabetes by causing your blood sugar level to rise.[1] How does this happen? Inorganic mercury or other toxic substance exposure can lead to essential mineral losses and gene dysfunction. When certain genes are not working properly, your body metabolism changes. Changes in body metabolism can result in the development of type 2 diabetes or other diseases associated with the Western diet. What you eat determines how your genes behave. That is why you need access to a food supply that is not contaminated with inorganic mercury or other toxic substances. In writing this book, I hope to teach you the difference between a safe and unsafe food supply.

It is my belief that a safe food supply should not contain inorganic mercury or any other toxic element that has been shown to impact human health. I am not alone in this belief. For example, my view on inorganic mercury in the food supply is consistent with that of the American Academy of Pediatrics (AAP). The AAP recommends eliminating all mercury exposures from the child's environment, including from the diet.[2] The AAP also recommends removing certain mercury-containing food colors from a hyperactive or inattentive child's diet.[3] I agree with these recommendations! Mercury is a neurotoxin and has no place in our children's diets, despite the fact that it has been found in the most common food ingredient in the food supply by both American and Canadian researchers.[4,5]

There are many stakeholders involved in the food distribution system, and all have differing views on the safety of the food supply. Grocery manufacturers and food distributors are primarily concerned with extending product shelf life and increasing profits, while consumers are more concerned about food quality from a safety and health standpoint. Controversy surrounds foods grown with genetically modified organisms (GMOs) or with pesticides. This is why a growing number of consumers want their food labeled; they want to know what they are buying. In response to consumer demands, many grocery manufacturers are now voluntarily labeling food products with or without GMOs and pesticides. It is important to understand that consumers in some countries outside of the United States do not have to worry about the safety of their food supply because their governments have more power to regulate what goes into their food supply.

Some countries outside of the U.S. have banned the sale of grains grown with GMO seeds. This is because some of the science-based evidence tells us that growing GMO crops may lead to adverse environmental or human health impacts.[6] It is too early to determine if GMO crops are safe. Scientists cannot reach a consensus on the safety of foods grown with GMO technology.[6] What I do know is that in banning the sale of grains grown from GMO seeds, countries are taking a precautionary approach. It is better to be safe than sorry, because interpreting science-based evidence is tricky no matter what food or food ingredient we talk about. In the U.S., we do not take this precautionary approach in regulating the use of chemicals, GMO seeds, or food ingredients.[7] The European Union (EU), on the other hand, *does* take a precautionary approach in regulating chemicals, including those used to make food ingredients.[7]

For example, in EU countries, the use of certain food color ingredients must be accompanied with a warning label to consumers.[8] Some food colors are even banned from use in food in these countries. These food colors are so heavily regulated because studies have shown these colors may cause hyperactivity in children.[9,10,11] It is important for you to understand there is inequality among countries in the treatment of food safety issues and the regulation of food ingredients. This indirectly impacts disease prevalence.

The purpose of this book is to shed some light on the issues related to food safety in the U.S. and elsewhere. It is my belief that every consumer has a right to learn what is known or not known about the safety of our food supply. If you are a parent, this knowledge is especially important for the health of your children. The Standard American Diet (SAD) is comprised of many unsafe food ingredients that impact the way your genes function, leading to the development of common Western diseases such as heart disease and diabetes. I am writing this book because there is a need to educate consumers about the quality of the food supply so they can make the best decisions for their families when they are shopping for food at the grocery store. In this book, I take an inside look at the food manufacturing industry's practices and history, and how these have shaped our diets and health today. It is my hope that you will join me in the pursuit of an honest food regulation industry and a safe food supply.

Food safety is a problem for most families in the United States, rich or poor, whether they know it or not. I know this for a fact because I have studied the SAD extensively, published my findings with collaborators in peer-reviewed medical journals,[1,4,12,13] and for many years worked at the agency responsible for food safety in the U.S.—the Food and Drug Administration (FDA).

Introduction

This book is about creating a food supply in your home that is safe and free of toxic substances. These toxic substances include heavy metals (such as mercury) and pesticides. Using scientific research and my own experiences, I illustrate how such substances (as well as our diets in general) are contributing to Western diseases like diabetes, heart disease, Alzheimer's disease, autism, and more. Most of the public has no idea that the food they eat may contain these substances because of loopholes in the laws, misleading food product labels, and faulty risk assessment processes. I know this because of the research I conducted—and then was ordered to *stop* conducting—during my time as an employee of the Food and Drug Administration (FDA).

I transferred to the FDA in 1999 as a Public Health Service (PHS) officer from the United States Environmental Protection Agency (EPA). My job at both the EPA and FDA involved the identification, assessment, mitigation, and cleanup of toxic elements left behind on laboratory surfaces, in laboratory hood and ventilation systems, biosafety cabinets, and plumbing systems in research laboratories undergoing closure. At that time, my training and background was in environmental health and industrial hygiene. This means I was qualified to identify, assess, and control physical, chemical, biological, or other environmental hazards in the workplace or community that could cause injury or disease. While doing my job at the FDA, my collaborators and I kept finding mercury in the plumbing systems of laboratories undergoing closure. We wondered where it came from.

Fortunately, my supervisor at the FDA gave me permission to determine the source of the mercury contamination in the plumbing systems. During my investigation, I uncovered the unsettling fact that many laboratory chemicals contain mercury residue. When mercury is part of a molecular compound or in its elemental form, it is heavier than water and tends to settle at low points in plumbing systems.[1] Before environmental regulations were developed by the EPA for the disposal of hazardous waste, researchers just poured waste chemicals down the laboratory drains and the mercury settled in the sink traps and sumps. This is the reason why we kept finding mercury in the plumbing systems of the laboratories undergoing closure at FDA. You may wonder how the mercury residue got into the laboratory chemicals in the first place. I did, too.

THE SEARCH FOR MISSING MERCURY

I consulted with my peers working in the environmental field and asked if they knew how the mercury residue ended up in the laboratory chemicals. I interviewed a colleague at the EPA and found out the chlor-alkali chemical companies reported missing several tons of mercury from their manufacturing process every year to the EPA.[2] (Chlor-alkali is a chemical process used to manufacture many industrial substances.)

In 2000, the twelve mercury cell chlor-alkali plants in operation at the time reported to EPA that there were approximately 65 tons of missing mercury altogether.[2] This amount was the difference between how much mercury the plants used and how much mercury the plants released into the environment or disposed of. The chemicals manufactured by the chlor-alkali plants were often the same ones used by FDA research laboratories.

My EPA colleague informed me that there was only one mercury cell chlor-alkali chemical company that had provided the EPA with information on where their missing mercury went. Out of the nine mercury cell chlor-alkali chemical companies operating in 2004, Vulcan Chemical was the only one in the United States to achieve its goal of finding its missing mercury. Vulcan Chemical knew exactly how much mercury went into their manufacturing processes to make chlorine, hydrochloric acid, sodium hydroxide, and potassium hydroxide chemical products, and where the mercury ended up. I suspected much of it ended up in the chemical products that the FDA and other researchers used in their laboratories, but needed to investigate further to see if my hunch was correct. I figured it would be best to go to the source, and so I telephoned Vulcan Chemical. No one was available to talk with me. I left a message for management staff, but they did not return my call.

The Vulcan Chemical mercury cell chlor-alkali manufacturing plant was located in Wisconsin, and I knew the company would have been required to comply with state environmental laws pertaining to toxic substance releases in wastewater and air. I submitted a request to the Wisconsin Department of Natural Resources (DNR) for information regarding the missing mercury from the Vulcan Chemical plant. The exact amounts were provided to me in an email from a wastewater specialist in the Wastewater Permits and Pretreatment Section.[3] Vulcan Chemical had provided this information to the DNR as part of their wastewater discharge permit application. The information is provided in the box below:

Missing Mercury (Hg) Found in Vulcan Chemical Products in 1999

- *Chlorine (Cl).* 1 lb Hg/year.
- *Sodium Hydroxide/caustic soda (NaOH).* 6 lb Hg/year.
- *Hydrochloric Acid/muriatic acid (HCl).* 11 lb Hg/year.
- *Potassium Hydroxide/potash (KOH).* 11 lb Hg/year.

As you can see in the box above, 1 pound of the missing mercury was found in the chlorine product, 6 pounds were found in the sodium hydroxide, and 11 pounds were found in both the hydrochloric acid and the potassium hydroxide. I realized at this point that mercury residue would probably be found in all chemical products produced by the mercury cell chlor-alkali industry. Since the mercury was missing from this industry, obviously no one had been keeping track of it. This fact alarmed me greatly because mercury is known to be extremely toxic among public health professionals. It is a neuro-toxin, which by definition interferes with brain development. What if the missing mercury ended up in products consumed by children? I knew the American Academy of Pediatrics had published a paper recommending the elimination of all mercury exposure from our children's environment.[4] The question that came to my mind was: Who else uses these mercury cell chemical products, besides scientists working in research laboratories?

I didn't have to look far for an answer to this question. It was lurking on the Vulcan Chemical website. Mercury-grade sodium hydroxide and hydrochloric acid were chemicals used primarily by the food color, citric acid, and high fructose corn syrup industries. Why would manufacturers use these mercury-containing chemicals to make food ingredients? Maybe the corn syrup manufacturers would talk with me. After all, I worked at the FDA.

MERCURY AND HIGH FRUCTOSE CORN SYRUP

The only corn refiner I could find who was willing to speak with me was the manager of an "organic" high fructose corn syrup (HFCS) manufacturing plant. The gentleman informed me that while the HFCS industry used both mercury cell sodium hydroxide and mem-brane grade sodium hydroxide in their manufacturing process to lengthen and enhance product shelf life, the mercury cell sodium hydroxide was preferred when it was available. I asked him if I could send out an FDA field investigator to collect samples of HFCS for mercury analysis and he said yes, as long as I agreed to keep his iden-tity confidential. He was alarmed at the possibility there could be mercury residue in his product as a result of using mercury cell sodium hydroxide in his manufacturing process and wanted to be cooperative.

I was alarmed that mercury cell sodium hydroxide was even allowed to be used in the HFCS manufacturing process in the first place. That year (2004), Americans were consuming 36 pounds of HFCS per person, which seemed like a lot of sweetener to me—especially when the substance could be contaminated with mercury.[5]

I contacted someone at the Chlorine Institute, the trade association that represented the chlor-alkali chemical manufacturers, to find out why food manufacturers could buy and use their mercury cell chemical products.

The president of the Chlorine Institute at the time, Art Dungan, was most cooperative and provided me with information on the allowable levels of mercury in "food grade" chlor-alkali chemicals.[6] He explained the amount of mercury residue in mercury cell chlor-alkali products varies, depending on the manufacturing process at each plant.[6] Manufacturers of mercury cell chlor-alkali chemicals are required to provide information regarding the amount of mercury found in their products on their product specification sheets.[6] Mr. Dungan explained the allowable levels of mercury and lead in food grade chemicals are established by the Food Chemicals Codex, the internationally recognized food ingredient safety standards, now owned and published by U.S. Pharmacopeial Convention (otherwise known as the USP).[7]

After doing some digging, I learned the USP was founded in 1820, long before the FDA, and is essentially the trade association for the pharmaceutical industry.[8] According to the Vulcan Chemical web page, the two largest purchasers of its mercury cell chlor-alkali chemicals were the pharmaceutical and high fructose corn syrup manufacturers! It appeared to me that mercury residue was purposely being added to both medicines and food ingredients. Why? What do food and medicine have in common?

Further research revealed mercury has historically been used as a biocide in medicines designed to kill germs or other pathogenic organisms, and as a pesticide in chemical products designed for killing mold on seeds and grains.[9] In medicine, it was incorporated in de-worming agents, teething powders, and diaper rash creams.[9] Prior to being taken off the market, Mercurochrome (an antiseptic containing mercury) was used routinely to treat sore throats and prevent infection in wounds.[9] In fungicides, mercury was an element used in agents designed to kill mold in and on grains.[10] Mercury compounds were used extensively in agriculture and in food production.[10]

The purpose of using mercury cell chlor-alkali chemicals to manufacture food ingredients is clear to me now. It makes sense that mercury residue in any food ingredient would kill mold and bacteria and lengthen product shelf life. The longer a product stays fresh on the grocery shelf without spoiling, the better for food manufacturers because product losses are minimized and profits are maximized, increasing net earnings. I became increasingly aware of how many food products contained high fructose corn syrup. I still could not believe mercury-containing chlor-alkali chemicals were intentionally being added to HFCS during the manufacturing process to enhance product shelf life. I wondered if HFCS manufacturers were touting their food ingredient's ability to prevent food product spoilage by killing bacteria or mold.

A quick visit to the Corn Refiner Association's web page revealed high fructose corn syrup was indeed being marketed as an ingredient capable of enhancing product shelf life by "creating freshness," or allowing manufactures to produce foods that stay fresh.[11] After viewing manufacturer's and distributor's websites, I read about how HFCS could be added to bread to "prevent mold." Some websites even touted the ingredient's use as a preservative. It was not approved by FDA for use as a preservative. How much mercury was in this ingredient, anyway?

To find out, I asked an FDA field investigator to visit a number of high fructose corn syrup manufacturers and collect samples for analysis. These samples were sent to a researcher's laboratory at a different agency that had analytical equipment that could detect the lowest levels of mercury; they were then placed in cold storage for safekeeping. I obtained another set of samples directly from the manufacturers and sent them to an analytical chemistry lab at the National Institute of Standards and Technology (NIST) and a University of California laboratory for analyses.

The researchers at NIST analyzed the HFCS samples and found trace amounts of mercury in all of them, as did the researchers who analyzed the samples at the University of California laboratory. It was time to report my findings to the FDA Center for Food Safety and Applied Nutrition (CFSAN). The University of California researcher sat in at the meeting with CFSAN staff and together, we reported the findings. To my amazement, after the meeting, I was ordered by senior FDA management to stop my investigation. Later, when I tried to publish the findings provided to me in an official report by the researchers at NIST,[12] I was informed by FDA management staff that I could not use the results in the official NIST report because they were not meant for "public distribution."

It became increasingly clear to me that in order to finish the investigation and report the findings, I would have to retire early from the Public Health Service. As a commander in the Public Health Service, if I disobeyed the direct order to "stop investigating," I could be prosecuted under the Uniform Code of Military Justice. Since I would not be allowed to continue the investigation, I asked my supervisor if I could tell the researcher who was safekeeping those HFCS samples sent to him by the FDA field investigator to do whatever he wanted with them. To my relief, my supervisor said yes. I immediately made plans to retire early to continue the investigation and find out the truth about the use of mercury as a preservative in our food supply.

MY MISSION

Since my retirement, I have continued the investigation with collaborators at research institutions and universities throughout the United States. We publish our findings in peer-reviewed medical journals. Now, I serve as the founding director and principal investigator at the Food Ingredient and Health Research Institute (FIHRI), the only federally-recognized 501(c)(3) nonprofit organization in the United States devoted entirely to food ingredient safety, consumer education, and research.[13,14] There is no other organization in the U.S. devoted to conducting research on food ingredients, such as HFCS, that are generally recognized as safe by the FDA. There are numerous food additives and ingredients recognized as safe by the FDA in our food supply that recent research indicates are factors in the development of autism, attention deficit-hyperactivity disorder (ADHD), and chronic diseases such as obesity and diabetes.

This book is a compilation of the research findings conducted by FIHRI, U.S. government scientists, and other researchers at universities across the world, written in consumer-friendly terms. This is combined with my knowledge and experience of working at a federal food regulation agency, the FDA. The research on food ingredients to date is science-based and the findings described for you here will guide you in creating a safe food supply for your family.

In Chapter 1, you will be introduced to the most common toxic substances that end up in our food supply. The guidelines that are used to assess the risk of such substances is problematic, and this chapter will explain why. In Chapter 2, you will learn how your genes function, their important roles in maintaining your health, and how they respond to what you eat. Chapter 3 discusses pesticide exposures in food and how they create conditions for adult-onset diseases. In Chapter 4, I will discuss food ingredients that can contain heavy metals, such as vegetable oils and corn sweeteners, and how they affect your current and future health status. Chapter 5 defines the Standard American Diet (SAD), which is sorely lacking in certain nutrients that help prevent disease.

Chapter 6 sheds light on the autism and ADHD epidemics and provides guidance to parents on what they can change in their family diet to alleviate the behaviors associated with these disorders. In Chapter 7, I will briefly outline the history of food safety regulation in the U.S. and describe the relationship between food manufacturers and the federal government. You will also learn how to read food ingredient labels so you can choose the safest products and foods to buy at the grocery store without falling for misleading claims. Finally, in Chapter 8, I will provide tips for creating and maintaining a safe food environment at home. It may seem impossible to avoid toxic substances in your food, but if you are armed with the information you need, you will find it is not so hard—and you and your family will feel healthier as a result.

By the time you are finished reading the Conclusion at the end of this book, I hope you will be able to apply what you learn to your family's daily life and improve the quality of food you serve at your dinner table. In creating a nutritionally adequate and safe food supply for your family members, you will not only enhance their quality of life, but also improve their chances of remaining healthy during their life span.

1.

What Are
Toxic Substances?

Imagine you are listening to a news broadcast about a food recall, or you are discussing with some friends a post you read online about chemicals found in baby food. You may have heard the word "toxic" brought up in these conversations about food safety. However, the specifics of this term are rarely defined. What makes a substance toxic? In what ways are these substances dangerous, and how do they become incorporated into your food? Because consumers are often unaware of the level of toxic substances that can be found in food, they may be ingesting metals (such as mercury) that have found a way into their favorite snacks. Some consumers may have knowledge about toxic substances, but underestimate the effects that even trace amounts can have on their health.

This book has been written to raise awareness for anybody who wants to create a safe food supply for himself or for his family. In this chapter, you will learn how a substance may become toxic, which is just another word for "harmful," as well as how such substances can enter your food via processing chemicals. We will discuss the state of science with respect to the measurement of toxic substances in blood and body fluids. We will discuss the change in the thinking about exposure to toxic substances that has occurred over the last few years. You will learn about the paradigm shift that has taken place in the United States and Europe in conducting research on toxic substances.

WHAT MAKES A SUBSTANCE TOXIC?

Any substance can be toxic or harmful to human health depending on the circumstances. Even something as common as caffeine can become toxic if it is consumed in a higher amount than the body can handle; if this happens, you may experience caffeine overdose and become seriously ill. Caffeine occurs naturally in many plants, including coffee beans, tea leaves, kola nuts (used to flavor cola soft drinks), and cacao pods (used to make chocolate).[1] It can also be man-made and added to foods, drinks, and medicines.[1]

When caffeine is added to a food, it must be included on the list of ingredients on the food product label and may not exceed 200 parts caffeine per million parts food product (ppm).[2] Under normal circumstances, consuming moderate amounts of caffeine is not harmful.[1] People with liver or heart disease, however, can die from caffeine intake, even at levels well below what is normally considered toxic.[3] The United States Food and Drug Administration (FDA) cited the case of a college student who died after taking too many caffeine pills to stay awake.[1]

Please note that although death by caffeine overdose is rare, this example illustrates how there has been a shift in thinking throughout the years regarding the concept of a toxic substance. The definition of a toxic substance should no longer be limited to heavy metals and pesticides, although these substances make up the majority of this book's subject matter because of their prevalence in food processing and their potential for causing harmful disease conditions. A toxic substance can be *any* item that causes you harm when it is consumed in amounts higher than what your body can handle (which, for some substances, is *any* amount).

Additionally, what is toxic to one person may not be toxic to another due to gene variability. The venom from a bee sting is annoying to somebody who is not allergic, but toxic to a person who *is* allergic.[4] Such a person can die within minutes from a single sting; his airway becomes swollen and he can no longer breathe, or his heart stops beating.[4] Individuals can have a life-threatening allergic reaction when exposed to a specific food ingredient or types of food; you probably know someone who is allergic to peanuts.

The important lesson here is that—much like caffeine—a food ingredient can become a toxic substance depending on the circumstances. Toxic substance exposure may cause harm immediately, or within a few seconds, minutes, hours, days, or many years down the road.

The FDA recommends that a healthy adult consume no more than four or five cups of coffee, or 400 mg of caffeine, a day.[5] FDA has not set a safe level for caffeine consumption for young children and adolescents,[5] although the substance continues to be "generally recognized as safe" (GRAS) and is being added to a growing number of food products.[5,6] (We will discuss the GRAS list in more detail in Chapter 7.)

In addition to energy drinks, caffeine is reportedly now being added to chewing gum, jelly beans, marshmallows, sunflower seeds, and other snack foods.[5] In 1978, some FDA scientists recommended that caffeine lose its GRAS status because the long-term, or chronic, effects of caffeine exposure in children and adolescents were unknown.[6] The scientists suggested there was a need to conduct human studies so the risk of adverse effect from long-term caffeine exposure could be determined and appropriate guidelines for exposure could be set for children and adolescents.[6] To date, these studies have not yet been done.

Guidelines for safe levels of caffeine—or any other toxic substance exposure—cannot be determined until appropriate studies have been conducted and a formal risk assessment process has been undertaken by government agencies (see "Risk Assessment and 'Safe' Substances" on page 12). If there are no studies available to support the development of a guideline for allowable exposure to a given substance, then—under the current system of risk assessment—the substance is deemed "safe." Such is the case with caffeine as an added ingredient in food products. However, this sort of system is flawed because the toxicity of a substance cannot be defined by an exposure limit. Toxic substance exposure that is below a government limit does not necessarily mean the exposure is safe and harmless. The "upper limit" is a misleading guideline that disguises the fact that some substances found in processed foods should not be consumed *at all*. (See page 13 for more information about upper limit levels.) Throughout

"Toxin" versus "Toxicant"

Throughout this book, we discuss man-made toxic substances that have been found in food. These toxic substances include organophosphate pesticides and heavy metals like mercury. You have likely heard these substances be incorrectly referred to as *toxins*. However, *toxins* are the natural substances produced by a plant or animal. When discussing man-made substances, such as the ones discussed in this book, the correct word to use is *toxicant,* which is another word for "toxic substance." The word "toxin" will not be used in its place.

this book, we will discuss such toxic substances, including heavy metals and organophosphate pesticides.

Note that the proper term for man-made toxic substances such as these is *toxicant,* not *toxin.* (See inset "'Toxin' versus 'Toxicant'" above.)

Risk Assessment and "Safe" Substances

An upper limit exposure guideline for a substance usually comes from a review of the published studies (literature), which occurs during the *risk assessment* process. Risk assessment is the formal process used to estimate *risk*—the nature and probability of adverse health effects in humans who may be exposed to a given substance now or in the future.

If there is no literature available to support the development of a guideline for allowable exposure to a given substance, then—under the current system of risk assessment—the substance is deemed "safe."

However, some "safe" substances may contain unsafe elements. Take the example of water. You have no doubt heard stories of the most common contaminants in drinking water—lead and arsenic. Both of these elements are considered "heavy metals" because they are at least five times denser than water.[7] The heavy metals arsenic, cadmium, inorganic mercury, and lead that can be found in our water and food supplies are considered systemic toxicants.[7] This means they have a high degree of toxicity because even at *low* levels of exposure, each element is known to cause multiple organ damage over time.[7] How heavy metal exposures become harmful involves many mechanisms, some of which are not clearly understood.[7] Each heavy metal takes its own molecular pathway to cause harm to health.

As we have seen, even an innocuous substance like water can become toxic over a period of several months or years if it is contaminated by one or more heavy metals. It is important to be cautious and knowledgeable about what you are consuming, especially if you are pregnant; a pregnant woman drinking water from a well containing naturally occurring arsenic may unknowingly expose her developing fetus to arsenic at levels above the recommended guideline. Toxic substance buildup in the womb can cause illness in children before they are even born. In later chapters, this book will review ways in which you can ensure the safety of your household's food and water supply. The risk assessment process cannot be entirely relied upon; it is not always a definite indicator of a substance's safety because there are so many variables. The "innocent until proven guilty" thought process does not work for risk assessment because so much of the incriminating evidence has yet to be discovered.

Upper Limits

In the case of food contaminants or other substances, a common guideline for allowable exposure is the upper limit (UL). Currently, a UL is defined as the maximum level of intake that is likely to pose no risk of harmful effect over a twenty-four-hour period. This is the amount of intake you can survive before becoming ill. The system we have in place does not determine ULs for all substances on the market, nor does it determine the conditions under which a substance is toxic to humans in every age group. The system does not determine *when*, or at what point, a substance will become lethal or harmful to a human being. There are no ULs established for peanuts or other allergens.

Government regulators try to establish safe levels of exposure for many other substances, but these levels do not consider the toxic effects that may occur over time, especially in sensitive populations such as the developing fetus, children, and the elderly. The risk assessment system is flawed because there are too many variables that it does not consider. It does not take into account all of the different circumstances that can surround the ingestion of a toxic substance. It does not consider excessive intakes that may occur over less than twenty-four hours or low levels of exposure to toxic substances that may occur over many months or years. Low levels of exposure to one or more substances over time can lead to harmful conditions.

Whenever a "safe" level of exposure is established for a given substance, what generally happens is the level of regulation will decrease over time. Meanwhile, science-based evidence accumulates

The Dangers of Fluoride

The U.S. Environmental Protection Agency (EPA) currently allows up to 4 milligrams of fluoride in each liter of drinking water, but since 2011, the EPA has been considering lowering this level due to the science-based evidence showing fluoride exposure over time may actually be quite harmful to sensitive populations.[8] In response to the new science-based evidence, the U.S. Public Health Service (PHS) recommends water districts not add fluoride to drinking water supplies if the natural levels of fluoride already exceed 0.7 mg/L.[9] You no doubt realize there is a big difference between 0.7 and 4 mg/L and may feel some concern about the fluoride levels in your own community's drinking water supply. (Please see the Resources section on page 163 for more information on water fluoridation.)

The continued disparity between the EPA and PHS recommendations on water fluoridation is remarkable, considering the controversy over fluoride safety has been ongoing for decades. Let me share with you the results of a review article published in the U.S. government's *Environmental Health Perspectives* journal in 2012. During the review, researchers examined the results of twenty-seven studies and determined that exposure to high levels of fluoride in the womb can impact child neurodevelopment[10]—specifically, children living in high-fluoride drinking water areas have significantly lower IQ scores than those children living in a low-fluoride area.[10] The researchers warned that much lower exposures could still cause detrimental harm to brain and shows the original "safe" level is no longer safe. Fluoride in drinking water is an excellent example (see "The Dangers of Fluoride" inset on page 14).

The bioaccumulation (buildup in our body tissues) of substances that become toxic over time and are of no use to the human body is one factor in the development of many modern disease conditions. There are many substances in the food supply that can accumulate in our blood and other body tissues and bring about toxic effects, leading to disease conditions. The air we breathe, the water we drink, and the food we eat are all sources of toxic substance exposure in the environment.

---

development in children, because rats exposed to 1 mg/L of fluoride in drinking water for one year showed significant changes in brain morphology compared with rats not exposed to fluoride.[10] (As rats are bigger than the developing human fetus, many scientists believe that whatever harms rats will harm the developing fetus and, by association, children.[11])

A UL, or maximum exposure limit, designed to protect *adults* from toxic effects will not protect the developing fetus, children, or other sensitive populations. Children and the developing fetus suffer a disproportionate share of the adverse effects of water fluoridation.

But what about the elderly? When fluoride is ingested for many years, it is irreversibly and permanently incorporated into the bones.[12] Even when a drinking water supply contains only 1 mg/L fluoride, drinking that water will lead to the accumulation of 2,500 mg fluoride for each kilogram of bone in two years and 3,000–4,000 mg/kg over a lifetime.[12] Bone weakening begins at around 3,500 mg/kg.[12] Bone weakness from drinking fluoridated water is well-documented; more human studies correlate the 1 mg/L fluoride exposure level from drinking water with bone weakening than studies that do not.[12]

In other words, the evidence of harm associated with municipal water supply fluoridation is overwhelming. The body has no use for fluoride, which effectively displaces calcium in bone tissue, leading to conditions such as osteoporosis and heart disease.[12] Fluoride has no nutritive or physiologic value.[12] It only causes harm as time goes on.

In this book, our main concern is those substances that are not safe at any level, yet are used in the processing of many common foods. Although few studies have been conducted to determine the concentrations of heavy metals in food products, evidence suggests the most common toxic heavy metals found in the food supply are arsenic, cadmium, lead, and inorganic mercury.[13,14,15,16] As with fluoride (see page 14), these and many other elements and compounds—including those found in pesticides—that accumulate in our bodies have no significant role in keeping us healthy.

Although in this chapter we discuss heavy metal exposures, pesticide exposures are also contributing to the body's total burden of toxic substances. We will discuss pesticide exposures in detail in Chapter 3.

Arsenic

Arsenic is a metal, and exposure to it is linked with cancer, heart disease, infant mortality, skin lesions, lung cancer, and hampered immune function.[17] A worldwide health concern is the level of arsenic in drinking water. In 2001, the Environmental Protection Agency (EPA) lowered the acceptable level of arsenic in drinking water from 50 parts per billion (ppb) to 10 ppb.[17] However, the government has no way to enforce this limit on private well water.

Arsenic can be found in food due to the soil (arsenic can be used in pesticides), the water (arsenic can collect in the water runoff when it rains), and the food ingredient manufacturing processes. Rice, especially, is prone to arsenic exposure. The rice plants can extract arsenic from the soil in which they are grown.[18] A study was published in 2011 by scientists from Dartmouth College who tested the arsenic levels in the urine of pregnant women.[18] These scientists determined the arsenic exposures in the women that came from eating rice alone and from drinking water.[18] The women who ate rice had higher arsenic levels than the women who did not eat rice (5.27 μ/L versus 3.38 μ/L).[18] These findings are alarming, but do not mean you should not eat rice. Brown rice is a nutritious food and should be a part of a healthy diet, but it is important to find out its source (i.e., an organic farm or a farm that uses pesticides) and the method in which it is processed. This is part of creating a safe food supply at home.

These findings are especially relevant today; in a 2016 publication, scientists reportedly found adverse birth outcomes in pregnant women with higher arsenic levels.[19] The babies born to these women had significantly lower birth weights, smaller heads, and shorter lengths, compared with the babies born to women with lower arsenic levels.[19] What is even more relevant is the fact that arsenic exposure in the womb is linked to a depressed immune system and increased risk of lung cancer later in life.[19]

Cadmium

Cadmium is a highly toxic metal. It may be found in cigarette smoke, shellfish, liver meat, potatoes, or fish that have lived in cadmium-infested waters.[20] Cadmium is considered a *carcinogen,* meaning it is known to be a cause of cancer.[21] Other effects of exposure to high levels of cadmium include kidney disease, severe stomach pain, and vomiting.[21]

The FDA's maximum limit of exposure for cadmium in bottled water is .005 mg/L.[22] The FDA also allows up to 2 mg/L cadmium in certain food ingredients.[23] The body is slow to excrete this metal, so accumulation over a lifetime can occur depending on the consumer's metabolism.[24] Cadmium buildup can become toxic to the bones, much like fluoride (see page 14). This is mostly due to the effect cadmium has on calcium and vitamin D metabolism.[24] Additionally, when pregnant women are exposed to both cadmium and arsenic, there is a significant risk of congenital heart defect in the baby due to the co-exposures.[25]

Lead

Lead is a metal that is poisonous if inhaled or consumed. There is no safe level of exposure to lead.[26] Like fluoride, lead collects in our bones. It also targets the brain when it is found in the bloodstream.

Lead was a notable topic in the news in 2016 during the public health disaster in Flint, Michigan. In January 2016, President Barack

Obama declared a state of emergency when lead levels in water samples taken from the homes of Flint residents were found to contain up to 100 parts lead per billion parts water.[27] The current maximum amount of lead allowed in drinking water by the EPA is *zero*.[28] At the Hurley Medical Center near Flint, Michigan, pediatricians sounded the alarm when they found that children's blood lead levels had doubled during the public health crisis.[27] Studies conducted both in the distant past and more recently confirm that when blood lead levels are high, the lead impacts a child's ability to learn.[29] That is why EPA set the allowable exposure limit for lead in drinking water at zero. Ongoing exposure to lead is not acceptable under any circumstances.

In the elderly population, ongoing lead exposure is associated with the inability to differentiate between smells.[30] The *olfactory bulb,* located deep inside your nasal cavity, is the part of your brain that tells you what it is you are smelling. You can differentiate smells because your olfactory receptor cells communicate information to the olfactory bulb. Receptors are special brain cells that collect the incoming sensory information. Dysfunction of the olfactory bulb is an early warning sign of Alzheimer's disease.[30] Ongoing exposure to lead and other contaminants in water and food leads to the bioaccumulation of toxic substances in body tissues like the olfactory bulb, and is associated with serious brain and blood disorders.

Mercury

Like lead, mercury is a metal that is poisonous when ingested or inhaled. In the Preface of this book, I mentioned the extensive use of the mercury cell chlor-alkali chemical products (mercury cell sodium hydroxide/caustic soda, hydrogen chloride, potassium hydroxide, and chlorine) in food manufacturing processes. These chlor-alkali chemicals always contain mercury residues.[31,32,33] Caustic soda and hydrogen chloride are used routinely to regulate the acidity, or pH, of food products during manufacturing processes.[32] (The pH of food is regulated to preserve the food and prevent it from spoiling.) Current international food standards allow 1 microgram (µg) of mercury in each gram (g) of caustic soda used to process or manufacture food.[32,33] One µg/g is the same as 1 part per million (ppm).

There is no standard for mercury in food-grade hydrochloric acid, even though mercury contamination is likely.[34] The FDA considers hydrochloric acid to be generally recognized as safe (GRAS) for use as a neutralizing or buffering agent in food manufacturing processes.[34] (See Chapter 7 for more information on the GRAS list.) Mercury cell chlorine is also expected and allowed to contain a small amount of mercury residue; hence, there is an international standard for the amount of mercury in the chlorine used to bleach flour.[35]

So when you eat any food products, such as bleached flour, that are processed or made with the mercury cell chlor-alkali chemicals, you are at risk of inorganic mercury exposure. This inorganic mercury exposure adds to your body's burden of cumulative environmental exposures. In Chapter 4, I will go into more detail on the products that have been found to contain mercury residues or that are at high risk of mercury contamination. Inorganic mercury exposure is a concern because scientists have found that it will bioaccumulate in American blood[36,37] and may impact gene function and the body's ability to produce certain proteins.[37,38]

You may have heard that mercury can be in an organic or inorganic form. Organic mercury is simply mercury that is attached to one or more carbon molecules. Organic mercury molecules are most commonly found in fish and the thimerosal used to preserve vaccines. The elemental, or inorganic, forms of mercury and lead are not attached to carbon, but they can attach to your tissues once they get inside your body in different ways, causing as much harm as when they are attached to carbon.

Mercury and other heavy metal exposures from eating processed foods are major factors in the development of many of the Western diseases. Throughout the remainder of this book, we will discuss the science-based literature that supports this view and the continued need for advances to be made through research and projects (see "Measuring Toxic Load" on page 22).

WHY ARE TOXIC SUBSTANCES DANGEROUS?

The metals that may be found in your food are toxic. But what do they do to your body, exactly? Over a lifetime, the levels of these substances gradually increase in your blood and tissues and can lead to critical illnesses. The reason for this is twofold. First, the majority of the foods in which these metals can be found are processed. The sheer amount of processed foods (and the lack of fresh, whole foods) Americans eat means that there are significant nutrient deficits in the bodies of both children and adults. These deficits contribute to many Western diseases, such as diabetes, and neurological disorders, such as autism or ADHD.

Second, exposure to toxic metals interferes with gene function, which you will learn more about in Chapter 2. The types of genes that are affected are important for metabolizing and eliminating harmful substances from the body. When these genes are not functioning the way they should be, brain function deteriorates.

Some of the conditions that are associated with toxic substance exposure are:

- ADHD
- Autism
- High blood pressure (hypertension)
- High blood sugar (hyperglycemia)
- Cardiovascular (heart) disease
- Diabetes
- High cholesterol
- Obesity

We will go into more detail on this topic in Chapters 5 and 6.

TAINTING THE FOOD SUPPLY

With all of the possible adverse effects associated with metals such as lead and mercury, how do these substances end up in common foods? Next time you are in the supermarket, check out the ingredient lists on packaged foods. You will probably see ingredients such as high fructose corn syrup, vegetable oil, or food coloring (e.g.,

Yellow 5). In Chapter 4, we will provide details as to how heavy metals end up in these ingredients. However, there is some basic information you need to know first. There are some chemicals that are used extensively to manufacture food ingredients.[39] These chemicals include chlorine, hydrogen chloride, and sodium hydroxide. You will *not* see them on the food ingredient label, but they are there nonetheless, lurking inside the product. Their potential for harm is acknowledged by few.

Chlorine

If you've ever been in a swimming pool, you are probably already familiar with chlorine. It is the chemical used to disinfect and sanitize the pool. When combined with outside contaminants that swimmers bring into the pool, chlorine gives off a distinctive, strong scent. The bleach in your laundry room may also contain chlorine. You may be surprised to learn that this harsh cleanser is also used in food processing, mostly to bleach flour.[40] Mercury cell chlorine is expected and allowed to contain a small amount of mercury residue, and there is an international standard for the amount of mercury in flour-bleaching chlorine—1 ppm.[35] If you want to limit your and your family's mercury exposure, it is best to avoid food products containing the ingredients "bleached flour" or "bleached wheat flour."

Hydrogen Chloride

Hydrogen chloride, also known as hydrochloric acid, is used to regulate the acidity (pH) of food. As a "generally recognized as safe" (GRAS) substance, it can be used without limit in food manufacturing.[34] If it is made with the mercury cell process, hydrogen chloride will always contain mercury residues. Due to its unlimited use in food manufacturing processes, this substance is of particular concern; this is because the FDA did not consider the potential mercury residues that may be found in it when the agency conducted its risk assessment in 1979.[41] (As you learned on page 14, one of the problems with the risk assessment process is that once an upper limit of a substance is determined, further regulation of that substance tends to fall off. The public would certainly benefit from another, more recent risk assessment of hydrogen chloride.)

According to the FDA, hydrogen chloride is not a risk when used in food processing, or as a food additive to adjust the pH, because it is neutralized or buffered by the food to which it is added.[41] In determining the risk of harm to health, FDA wrote, "The small amounts of hydrochloric acid that may persist in foods or drinks, would, in turn, be neutralized and buffered during ingestion and digestion, or after absorption."[41] The potential presence of inorganic mercury in hydrogen chloride was completely ignored by the FDA in their opinion and thus, its potential as a source for mercury exposure was ignored in the risk assessment.

Sodium Hydroxide

Like hydrogen chloride, sodium hydroxide (also called caustic soda or lye) is used to regulate the acidity (pH) of food. For example, it is added to older, degraded vegetable oils to remove free fatty acids.[42] These acids are removed to enhance the value and taste of the oils; otherwise, there would be a bitter or rancid flavor in food products that contain these vegetable oils.[42] As mentioned on page 19, 1 ppm of mercury is allowed in this chemical. The small amount of sodium hydroxide that is added to vegetable oils could be a significant source of inorganic mercury exposure when we consider that the average American consumed 36 pounds of vegetable oil in the year 2012 alone.[43] Food preservation and product shelf life are important problems for food manufacturers to address, but using mercury-tainted sodium hydroxide is not the right answer.

MEASURING TOXIC LOAD

You may be wondering how you can find out for sure if you have ingested toxic substances. University research laboratories are working on perfecting the technology used to measure the amount of harmful substances in your blood. Unfortunately, the modern commercial medical laboratory has not yet been able to adopt the newest technologies. The typical commercial lab is not set up and able to measure with complete accuracy the body's total burden (load) of all the toxic substance exposures we are getting from the food we eat.

Biomarker Testing on
Blood, Hair, Fingernails, and Urine

A *biomarker* is a biological substance that can be measured using laboratory tests or instruments. Biomarker measurements can help doctors determine the presence or absence of disease and whether environmental exposures have taken place. Commercial medical laboratories can perform tests on different body fluids or tissues to determine the various biomarker levels associated with toxic substance exposure, such as mercury, lead, and pesticides. For example, if you had symptoms of organophosphate (OP) pesticide exposures (such as headache, fatigue, gastroenteritis, anxiety, and memory issues) and wanted to determine whether or not your body was being overburdened with these kinds of compounds, you could ask your doctor for an order to run a red cell *cholinesterase*.[44]

Cholinesterase is an enzyme the body produces to maintain its nervous system function. The levels of this biomarker in red blood cells can determine your exposure to the common organophosphate pesticides found in many grain products. OP pesticides, mercury, lead, and cadmium all inhibit or suppress cholinesterase production.[45] If your body is exhibiting symptoms of OP pesticide or heavy metal exposure, your cholinesterase levels will likely be low.[45] Cholinesterase testing is readily available through commercial medical laboratories.

Many medical laboratories can also measure total blood lead and mercury levels, but their equipment will not measure the smaller amounts of these elements or differentiate between all of the elemental forms that correspond to disease risk. Recall from page 19 that there are two forms of lead and mercury: Organic and inorganic. The organic substances are attached to carbon, while the inorganic forms are not. It is important to know that when laboratories measure the amount of mercury or lead in your blood, they are measuring *all* of the different forms of mercury and lead in your blood. Your laboratory blood mercury test result may read, for example, 3.25 µg mercury in

1 liter of blood (µg/L), but all this indicates is the *total amount* of mercury in your blood. The result does not tell you how much of the mercury is inorganic and how much is organic. The exact amount of each form of mercury will not be provided in the test result.

Commercial medical laboratories do not have the same capacity to measure toxic substances in body fluids as the universities doing research today; there is a disparity between the standard practices conducted in commercial medical laboratories today and the measurement capacity of university laboratories, where technological advances are being made.

Certain commercial medical laboratory instruments can only detect an element if it reaches a given level in a body fluid. This level is called the "detection limit." The good news is that there are commercial laboratories that have developed the technology to measure lower levels of elements and compounds associated with disease risk. Soon there will be the capacity to not only measure individual elements and compounds at low levels, but also determine the individual's cumulative risk of disease based on *all* of their test results and what is now known in the available literature. The science is only about two to five years ahead of the standard practice. In the Resources section of this book (found on page 163), you will find a list of laboratories that are actively engaged in the Human Exposome Project[46] (see section below).

The Human Exposome Project

The Human Exposome Project is an international effort to determine how cumulative environmental exposures lead to various diseases. The project is funded by both the U.S. and European governments.[46] The *exposome* is a term used to describe the collective environmental exposure to contaminants that humans face over a lifetime. The Human Exposome Project is based on a shift in thinking with respect to how diseases occur and what must be done to prevent them. Such a shift in thinking is called a *paradigm shift*. The Europeans were probably the first to embrace this paradigm shift because their medical care system is funded directly by their governments and based on disease prevention. Since before 2012, doctors in Europe have been working together to figure out how early-life exposures to multiple toxic substances in the womb contribute to child health outcomes.[47] The name of the European exposome project is HELIX.[47]

In 2013, the U.S. government funded the country's first and only exposome research center at Emory University in Atlanta, Georgia by providing a $4.5 million grant to be used over four years.[48] The name of the center is HERCULES, and it operates with considerably less focus than HELIX.[49] As a researcher who has investigated the role of toxic substances in the food and water supply on adverse birth outcomes and the development of type 2 diabetes, I am not impressed with the projects that have been funded thus far by HERCULES.

For example, the HERCULES projects being researched in 2016 are not focusing on dietary exposures to substances that will become toxic over time or that impact human development and lifespan. The projects do not address the maternal nutritional factors that may improve overall health outcomes of the children being born today. Whether you have children or not, the future of America rests on the intellectual capacity of children born today and their perspective lifelong health outcomes. Everyone begins life in the womb; the diet of a pregnant woman and what she later feeds her child determines that child's capacity for learning and whether he will suffer from type 2 diabetes later in life or die of heart disease. Every American should be concerned about our society's children. They are our capital asset and we must reduce their exposures to toxic substances to ensure the best health and learning outcomes. It is my hope that by the end of this book you will see why this is so important.

CONCLUSION

I believe the majority of our toxic substance exposures comes from the food we eat and the water we drink. Substances (such as fluoride) may be deemed safe at certain levels by the FDA and EPA, but once they enter our bodies, they accumulate in our blood and tissues or impact the way our genes function to alter our body metabolism. They become toxic over time. Such substances also include the chloralkali chemicals—such as chlorine, hydrogen chloride, and sodium hydroxide—that contain mercury residues and are used to make food ingredients, manufacture food products, and process agricultural commodities. In addition to mercury, other heavy metals that contaminate the food supply and drinking water are arsenic, cadmium, chromium, and lead. Pesticide residues are also found widely in agricultural commodities. These residues contribute to our bodies' total burden of toxic substance load exposure and are associated with the development of disease. Without evidence of harm, substances are presumed to be safe, and no exposure guidelines are developed. Safe levels of exposure to toxic substances may only be determined after a number of human studies have been conducted and a formal risk assessment process has been undertaken by government agencies.[50]

I hope that by now, this discussion has led you to an understanding of how a substance can be or become toxic. You have learned that a toxic substance is not always labeled in a bottle illustrated with a skull and crossbones. Even a widely consumed substance, like caffeine, can become toxic if consumed in amounts higher than what your body can handle. There are numerous mechanisms or pathways for substances to cause harm in the body; we will explore some of these in later chapters. One of the most important mechanisms involved in the development of disease is gene function, which will be the subject of the next chapter.

2.

Genes and Your Health

I n Chapter 1, you were introduced to the toxic substances that can find their way into your food supply via processing chemicals. In this chapter, I will further explain how these substances affect your genes and, subsequently, your health.

The food you eat, the water you drink, and the air you breathe provide the fuel for your genes—the building blocks of your body. The substances you consume construct the *chemical compounds* that modify your genes' behavior. Changes in gene behavior affect your physical and psychological actions. In other words, gene function and behavior are directly related to health outcomes.

In this chapter, we will discuss genes and how they respond to the environment. For example, the quality of what your mother ate and drank and of the air she inhaled during pregnancy determined your health status today to a large degree. This does not mean that you cannot improve your health status. You can change your environment to improve your gene function and well-being. That is why it is so important to know the dangers of the toxic substances that are potentially in your food. In this chapter, we will clarify what genes are and what they do, and we will discuss how changes in diet can affect gene behavior over time.

WHAT DO GENES DO?

Genes are the units that give you your traits—for example, your eye color or hair color. Genes also determine your likelihood for developing specific conditions or illnesses. They provide the instructions that tell your cells what to do—in other words, they determine what a cell's job is going to be. For example, in the liver, there are different liver cells that do different things. In the blood tissue, there are different blood cells that do different things. The actions of these cells are managed by your genes.

Genes are made up of interconnected molecules called *nucleic acids*. "Nucleic" means these molecules are found in the nucleus of each cell. You've probably heard of DNA, or deoxyribonucleic acid. When people talk about DNA, they are really talking about your genes (your genes are made up of DNA). Genetic material in the human *genome* (the complete set of genes in a person) is made up of approximately 21,000 genes comprised of the nucleotide structures found in DNA (see inset "An Inside Look at DNA" on page 29). These genes are located in the chromosomes inside the nucleus of each cell. (See Figure 2.1 below for a visualization of where genes are located in your cells.)

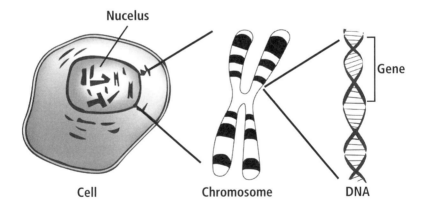

Nucelus

Cell **Chromosome** **DNA** **Gene**

Figure 2.1. The location of genes inside the cell.

We inherit our genes from our parents. Identical twins have the same set of genes in every single cell, but their genes will not necessarily behave the same way.[1] Specific genes "turn off" and "turn on." A process called *methylation* causes most of these changes. (See page 31.)

An Inside Look at DNA

DNA is formed from nucleic acid structures called *nucleotides.* Each nucleotide consists of a phosphate, sugar, and one nitrogen base molecule. There are four base molecules: Adenine (A), cytosine (C), guanine (G), and thymine (T). A nucleotide can be made with any one of the four bases. Your genes are made up of a series of nucleotide structures joined together in a special way when the bases pair up with one another. Individual genes vary in size and can be made up from a few thousand to over 2 million base pairs.[2] The bases always pair up the same way; adenine always pairs with thymine and cytosine always pairs with guanine. These paired bases will vary in sequence, as the structure of the DNA molecule differs between individuals. The DNA in a human egg or sperm cell is comprised of several *billion* base pairs. The innumerable possible DNA sequences is the reason why no two people in the world are exactly the same. The picture below is simplified, but will give you an idea of the structure of DNA.

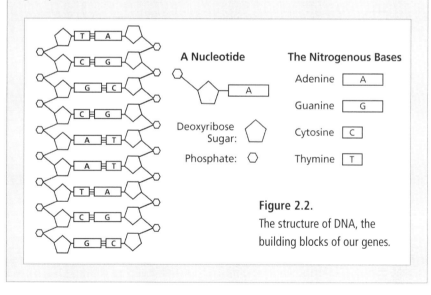

A Nucleotide

The Nitrogenous Bases

Deoxyribose Sugar:

Phosphate:

Adenine   A

Guanine   G

Cytosine   C

Thymine   T

Figure 2.2.
The structure of DNA, the building blocks of our genes.

Cell Differentiation

Cell differentiation is when a cell decides what kind of cell it will be and what it will do. No matter what genes you are born with, how they function inside your cells depends on the environment you create in your body. This is an important concept because gene function determines body function. For example, if you have a child with attention deficit hyperactivity disorder (ADHD), his genes are functioning in response to his environment. If you have developed type 2 diabetes, it is because your genes have responded to the environment you created in your body.

The study of how genes respond to or interact within their cellular environment is called *epigenetics.* This relatively new field of study is found in the biology discipline. "Epi" is a prefix that means "outside of" or "above" (see "Epigenetics" inset below).

Gene regulation occurs when chemical compounds are added to single genes, modifying their behavior; these modifications are known as *epigenetic changes.*[3] The food you eat, the water you drink, and the air you breathe provide the fuel and the individual atoms that construct these chemical compounds. All of the chemical compounds that regulate gene behavior make up what is known as the *epigenome.* How a human body functions is a direct result of the *epigenomic changes,* or modifications that remain as cells divide. The most common of these changes is called *methylation* (see "Methylation" on page 31). In some cases, these functional changes can be passed on from parent to child. For example, children with Asperger syndrome (considered a state of high-functioning autism) operate very much like their parents from both a psychological and anatomical perspective.[4,5,6] They inherited the way they function from their parents.

Epigenetics

"Epi" is a prefix meaning on, upon, outside of, or above. Approximately 330 words start with "epi." In this book, we will concern ourselves with the following words:

Epigenetics. Interactions occurring between genes and their environment.

Epigenome. All of the chemical compounds that regulate gene activity.

Epigenomic changes. Changes that occur as cells divide. These can be passed on from parent to child, or modified through dietary changes or exposure to toxic substances.

Methylation

Methylation is the most common type of epigenomic modification and involves the transfer of a methyl molecule, or "methyl group," to a gene.[3] A methyl group is made up of the elements carbon and hydrogen—specifically, one carbon atom and three hydrogen atoms (see Figure 2.3). When a methyl group is added to a gene, the gene may be turned "on" or "off" so that it is effectively silenced.[3] Once a gene is silenced, no protein can be produced from that gene.[3] The way methylation works is that proteins attach the methyl groups to the bases of the DNA molecule in specific places. In this way, cells can remember which genes are on or off. Your body needs these methyl groups to turn genes off and then back on again as needed.

The methyl group pictured in Figure 2.3 is sometimes referred to as a *hydrocarbon*. You can see the hydrogen atoms that are bonded, or attached, to the carbon atom.

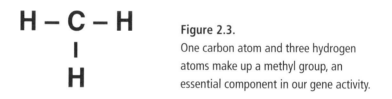

Figure 2.3.
One carbon atom and three hydrogen atoms make up a methyl group, an essential component in our gene activity.

Your body's ability to produce methyl groups is called *methylation*. The process of methylation continues throughout the human life span. If your body under-produces methyl groups, it is called *hypomethylation*. Hypomethylation occurs in children who have autism.[7,8] This means their bodies do not have enough methyl groups for use in carrying out bodily functions, and some of their genes are habitually turned off. Research has shown that these genes can be turned back on to produce the proteins needed by the child's body to significantly improve his language, communication, personal living skills, interpersonal social and coping skills, and overall behavior.[9] Switching these genes back on to improve the child's health requires more methyl groups for the methylation process.

How can these children obtain more methyl groups to switch the genes back on? It is a complicated process, but the food you eat is a factor in the production of methyl groups.[10,11,12] In your diet, methyl groups come from foods that contain methyl-donating nutrients such as methionine, choline, and folic acid (folate).[10,11,12] Diets deficient in methyl-donating nutrients will impact gene function via hypomethylation.[10] Epigenetic changes can occur in the womb, after a child is born, and throughout the child's life as a result of maternal and family diet.[13] Several diseases are associated with hypomethylation.[13,14,15,16] These include:

- Alzheimer's disease
- Atherosclerosis
- Autism
- Cardiovascular disease
- Hyperglycemia
- Hypertension
- Low high-density lipoprotein (HDL), the "good cholesterol"
- Type 2 diabetes

To prevent diseases of hypomethylation, you can increase your dietary intake of methyl-donating foods. I will provide a table of foods high in methyl-donating nutrients in Chapter 5.

THE IMPORTANCE OF GENES

Your genes contain the instructions for operating your body. This includes the prevention of certain diseases, such as Alzheimer's disease or type 2 diabetes. Your diet strongly influences how these genes function in your body. Here, we will focus on some of the most significant genes for your health, including oncogenes, PON1, and BDNF.

Oncogenes

Oncogenes are genes that cause cancer. What we are exposed to in our environment will determine how often our oncogenes will turn on. Viruses, toxic substances, and the sun's ultraviolet (UV) rays are examples of cancer-causing agents in the environment. We all have cancer cells in our bodies that must be destroyed by the proteins produced by our tumor suppressor genes. When these tumor suppressor genes turn on, the protein they produce encourages the death of cancer cells, effectively stopping their proliferation.

If an oncogene keeps turning on and won't stop expressing itself, you will develop a *tumor,* which is basically unregulated cell growth. For example, if you develop skin cancer, growths can appear on or under the skin and get larger as the skin cells continue to replicate uncontrollably. If the tumor does not grow quickly or invade other tissues, it will be classified as "benign." But everyone has the potential to develop a malignant tumor or cancer, because we all have oncogenes that are capable of expressing themselves uncontrollably.

In a healthy body, oncogenes are regulated by diet and nutrition. For example, scientists recently found that diet-influenced vitamin D status significantly affected the expression of 291 different genes, many of which were linked to cancer.[17] Not all of the genes reacted in the same way to vitamin D intake—some turned on and some turned off—but the data showed that any improvement in vitamin D status will improve the regulation of genes associated with cancer, cell differentiation, and immune function.[17]

BDNF

In addition to providing methyl groups and suppressing cancer-causing genes, your diet also provides your body the micronutrients it needs to build the proteins and enzymes expressed by the genes in your cells. For example, proteins that promote learning and enhance memory are produced by genes in your brain cells. *Brain derived neurotrophic factor* (BDNF) is an example of such a protein. It is produced by the BDNF gene.[18,19] You can think of the BDNF protein as the "glue" that attaches your memories to your brain cells.

BDNF gene regulation and BDNF protein production rely on both methylation and dietary calcium intake. BDNF gene expression levels are important in humans of any age. In a 2014 study, scientists determined BDNF protein levels in the blood of children with autism were significantly lower compared with the BDNF protein levels in healthy children of the same age.[20] Another group of researchers found that children with autism were less likely to eat foods providing adequate levels of calcium compared with healthy children, due to selective eating, a doctor- or parent-enforced restricted diet, or both.[21] What this means is children with autism generally eat fewer calcium-rich foods and have lower BDNF protein levels in their blood.

These exact same findings have been found in adults with Alzheimer's disease and other dementias.[22,23,24] To avoid dementia, you must ensure your diet is rich in calcium and methyl-donating groups so your brain cells can produce and express the BDNF protein needed to retain memories. People who become afflicted with Alzheimer's disease eventually will not be able to remember things such as math facts or the meaning of words in text.[25,26] Their diets will likely lack calcium and their BDNF genes will not be able to express enough protein to retain the memories of lessons learned from days gone by.

PON1

Another gene dependent on calcium for expression is *paraoxonase-1*, or PON1.[27] When it is expressed, it produces the enzyme paraoxonase, which is needed by your body to break down and metabolize the organophosphate pesticide residues found on and in various foods sold in American grocery stores.[28,29] Organophosphate (OP) pesticides are molecules that always contain carbon and phosphate atoms. Like any other substance, they can become toxic under certain circumstances.

The paraoxonase enzyme produced by the PON1 gene is crucial for breaking apart and destroying the OP pesticide molecules. These molecules must be broken down before they can be eliminated by the body.

PON1 enzyme is made by your liver cells and secreted in your blood, where it is incorporated into high density lipoprotein (HDL), or "good" cholesterol.[30] Inadequate dietary intake of calcium or the consumption of harmful food ingredients may impact PON1 gene expression.[28] Much like BDNF, the availability and activity of PON1 are impaired in many children with autism and adults with Alzheimer's and dementia.[28,31,32,33,34,35] PON1 enzyme levels are lower in these demographics.[31,33,34,35] Because evidence suggests that OP pesticide exposures are associated with the development of

Alzheimer's disease and dementia,[36,37] you may want to protect your future health by ensuring your dietary intake of calcium is adequate and reducing your dietary intake of harmful food ingredients. You will learn more about which food ingredients are considered harmful and which are helpful as we get further along in the book.

PON1 gene activity has been extensively studied in humans; there are a number of factors known to modulate, or alter, its expression. These factors include—but are not limited to—heavy metal exposure, sex, and age.[30,38] Age plays the most important role, as PON1 activity is very low before birth and through at least seven years of age.[38,39] PON1 activity is also lower in boys compared with girls.[30,38] This might explain why autism is more common in boys than girls, especially since autism is associated with OP pesticide exposures.[40]

In the elderly population, there is no significant difference between the incidences of Alzheimer's disease and dementia among men and women as they grow older.[41] Because PON1 activity is much lower in the elderly,[42,43] it is likely the reason why they are more susceptible to the neurotoxic effects of OP pesticide exposures.

Regardless of age, I recommend a diet rich in calcium and free of heavy metals to ensure your PON1 gene is functioning properly. Expectant mothers must be especially careful to ensure their dietary calcium intake is sufficient. In addition to supporting the activity of the BDNF and PON1 genes, calcium also helps to eliminate lead—one of the toxic heavy metals you read about in Chapter 1—from the body (see inset "Using Dietary Calcium to Eliminate Lead" on page 36). In Chapter 5, I will provide a list of foods that are high in calcium from the United States Department of Agriculture (USDA) National Nutrient Database.[44]

MT Genes

Metallothionein (MT) genes produce MT proteins, which are metal transporters. They perform a metal-clearing function in your body. These important MT proteins allow your body to excrete a number of toxic heavy metals, including mercury, copper, cadmium, lead, silver,

Using Dietary Calcium to Eliminate Lead

Children with ADHD and pervasive developmental delay (PDD) tend to accumulate lead—especially if their diets lack calcium—when they are exposed to lead in the environment.[45,46,47] Environmental lead exposure may occur in older homes painted with lead-based paint, or in contaminated drinking water (such as the 2016 case in Flint, Michigan, mentioned in Chapter 1). Water supplies anywhere may be impacted by lead in plumbing systems. Lead is also routinely found in air and soil. Lead exposure in the womb is now considered a risk factor for Alzheimer's disease.[48]

In the human body, lead and calcium atoms compete for the same "docking stations" on molecules, so if your diet is deficient in calcium, those docking stations will attract lead. By eating foods rich in calcium, you can help prevent the bioaccumulation of lead in your body tissues and support proper PON1 and BDNF gene expression.

and bismuth.[49] Scientists have published strong evidence that shows one cause of autism may be a result of a biochemical abnormality that disables the metal-clearing function of the MT proteins.[50,51,52,53] Other scientists have found that MT proteins are reduced in elderly people that have been diagnosed with Alzheimer's disease.[54] This reduction in MT protein levels could be an important factor in the underlying pathology of Alzheimer's.[55]

MT genes are dependent on zinc to produce the molecules that make up the MT proteins. Strong evidence shows that dietary zinc deficiency plays a role in Alzheimer's disease, autism, and ADHD.[54,55,56,57,58,59] If you are deficient in zinc or eating too much of a food ingredient that depletes zinc, then you may not be able to build the MT protein molecules needed by your body to excrete the heavy metals you are exposed to in the air you breathe and the food you eat.[49] When children with autism are zinc deficient and their MT genes are dysfunctional, their little bodies end up storing heavy metals that lead to neurological impairment.[51] Children with ADHD are also often zinc deficient, but there is no evidence to suggest they have MT dysfunction.

It is important to eat foods rich in zinc to prevent the bioaccumulation of neurotoxic heavy metals. In Chapter 8, I will provide a table with a list of foods that are high in zinc according to the USDA National Nutrient Database.[44]

HOW DIET AFFECTS GENES AND HEALTH

Throughout this chapter, you have read about what happens when certain genes turn "on" and "off." But what activates (or deactivates) these genes? A lot of the answer lies in nutrients. For example, you learned earlier in this chapter that foods containing methyl groups can turn genes on or off. Oncogene activity is quieted by vitamin D, while the beneficial activity of genes such as BDNF and PON1 rely on calcium. Some genes, such as the MT genes, are dependent on micronutrients other than calcium (e.g., zinc) for building their proteins.

The bioaccumulation of one or more heavy metals accompanies a number of Western diseases and neurodevelopmental disorders. *Pica* is the most common symptom exhibited by a person who is having difficulty excreting heavy metals. Such a person will often chew on objects such as ice, fingernails, or pencils, or compulsively eat particular foods or nonnutritive substances.[60] Children with pica may suffer from abdominal pain.[61] Complications of pica include lead and mercury poisoning.[60] Pica is associated with zinc deficiency, iron deficiency, and developmental delay.[60] It is a condition commonly found in children with autism and ADHD, but often under-diagnosed.[60,62,63,64] Pica can be under-diagnosed because most physicians are not trained in nutrition or toxicology.

Diets insufficient in zinc may compromise the body's ability to excrete the mercury and other heavy metals found in processed foods.[50] If the body is not able to rid itself of the inorganic mercury from processed food, it may become damaged in a number of ways as the mercury accumulates in the body. Inorganic mercury may prevent the activation of the PON1 gene in the liver, thus impairing the body's ability to protect itself against organophosphate pesticides.[38] This can result in the development of cardiovascular disease, Alzheimer's, chronic liver disease, chronic kidney disease, autism, or developmental delay.[30,31] Inorganic mercury may also alter glucose metabolism by suppressing the GLUT gene, which is responsible for regulating glucose levels.[65] This epigenetic change will then increase the risk of developing type 2 diabetes by elevating the blood sugar level.[65] As a result of nutritional deficiency, epigenetic changes may occur and impact the functioning of any one of the 21,000 genes in the human genome. (For more information on the human genome, see inset "The Human Genome Project" below.)

CONCLUSION

In this chapter, you have learned that dietary factors interact with genes to determine how your body functions. You learned about epigenetic changes, which occur when chemical compounds are added to genes and change their behavior. Diet plays an epigenetic role in gene function, first in the womb and then continuously and over a lifetime.[67] With advancing age, the food you eat can influence your chances of developing Alzheimer's disease, heart disease, hypertension, diabetes, autism, and other Western disease conditions. To

The Human Genome Project

The Human Genome Project is a research project that began in 1990 and was completed in 2003.[66] The project was financed by the U.S. government. The human genome of an egg or sperm consists of 3 billion base pairs of the four repeating bases, which can vary in sequence.[66] This sequence is the centerpiece of the Human Genome Project's research.

When an egg and sperm join together, an embryo is formed to start the creation of a new baby. As the fetus develops in the womb, each cell of its body will have two copies of unique genetic sequence, one from its mother and the other from its father. So, each cell in the baby's body will have 6 billion base pairs of DNA in the genetic material of the nucleus.[66] Growth is rapid in a developing fetus, baby, and child. With each cell division, there is the potential for epigenetic changes to occur that impact gene function, development, and health outcomes. Cells continue to divide over the course of the human lifespan.

protect yourself against these conditions, eat fresh, whole foods, especially ones high in methyl-donating groups, vitamin D, calcium, and zinc. These nutrients can enhance the genes that clear metals and pesticide residues from your body.

In addition to diet, environmental influences can impact gene expression. For example, pesticide exposure from inhalation of mists being sprayed by the farmer next door can cause epigenetic changes that impact a child's brain development. Exposure to organophosphate pesticides prior to and after birth is associated with the development of both autism and ADHD.[68,69,70,71,72,73,74] Pesticide exposures are also associated with the development of type 2 diabetes, heart disease, Alzheimer's disease, and Parkinson's disease. The focus of the next chapter will further discuss dietary pesticide exposures and their role in the development of adult-onset diseases.

3.

Pesticides and Adult-Onset Diseases

In the previous chapter, we reviewed how gene function or dysfunction impacts your health. Exposures to toxic substances in the environment or from the food we eat may impact the way certain genes function or create conditions of mineral loss that disrupt the body's ability to produce important proteins and enzymes. The inability to adequately produce certain proteins or enzymes may lead to adult-onset disease conditions such as type 2 diabetes, heart disease, or neurological disorders caused or made worse by pesticide exposures. In this chapter, we will discuss how pesticide exposures occur and their role in creating conditions for adult-onset disease. Before we begin, let's talk about what pesticides are, what they do, and why they are used to produce your food despite the risk of disease.

WHAT ARE PESTICIDES?

Pesticides are chemical compounds designed to kill specific pests, such as weeds or insects. Sometimes these pests can spread infectious diseases or bring destruction to the crops that are being raised for food.[1] There are many types of pesticides that serve different purposes. They are used on a variety of products—such as on wood to eliminate termites, or on cotton to kill bugs—but in this chapter, we will focus on the pesticides used on crops that are raised for food. Each pesticide contains an active ingredient that enables the compound to kill the target organism.

In the United States, the Environmental Protection Agency (EPA) regulates who gets to use the different pesticides and for what purpose. EPA-regulated pesticides can only be used by those who undergo pesticide applicator training and become certified (household products such as bleach or insect baits can be used by anybody). For example, chlorine compounds are regulated by the EPA for use as a disinfectant to kill bacteria and viruses and a fungicide to kill mold and other fungi[2] (see "An Inside Look at Chlorine" inset below). EPA allows your local water district to use chlorine (in a gas or in other forms) to treat the drinking water supply and the wastewater discharged from the sewage treatment plant. You may already be famil-

An Inside Look at Chlorine

Food manufacturers are authorized by the EPA to use chlorine as a "food rinse."[3] Substances like chlorine dioxide and sodium chlorite may be used on food or feed contact surfaces and on agricultural commodities.[3] These chlorine compounds are also routinely used at animal and poultry premises, including hatcheries (facilities in which eggs are hatched in artificial conditions).[3] The chlorine compounds may be applied on eggs and fresh fruits and vegetables post-harvest.[3] Interestingly, chlorine is one of the few pesticides allowed for use in organic food production and handling.[4] Organic farming typically restricts the use of synthetic (man-made) pesticides like chlorine.

The use of chlorine compounds in organic food production and handling is regulated by the U.S. Department of Agriculture (USDA), which provides specific guidelines to farmers.[4] The guidance states that "water used directly on crops or foods is permitted to contain chlorine at levels approved by the Food and Drug Administration or the Environmental Protection Agency for such purpose."[4] Remember, the chlorine compounds that farmers can add to water are considered pesticides. After the organic farmer uses the chlorinated solution on crops or foods, he must then triple-rinse the food with potable (drinkable) tap water.[4] The final rinse water may not contain more than the allowable levels of chlorine in drinking water.[4] The chlorine residue in drinking water is regulated by EPA. Because organic products are not allowed to

iar with chlorine as an ingredient in the bleach in your washing machine that helps white clothes stay white.

HOW PESTICIDE EXPOSURE HAPPENS

The problem with pesticide use is that when we use these com-pounds, we will become exposed to them, especially when we eat conventionally grown crops or live near agricultural operations. Pesticide use isn't just the practice of spraying fields and crops with EPA-regulated neurotoxins. For example, the organophosphate (OP) pesticide *malathion* is applied directly on grain in storage silos

contain pesticide residues, the rinsing process described here is the rea-son you will see the words "triple-rinsed" on packaging that contains organic produce.

EPA has admitted that there are chronic exposures to chlorine occurring in the population from the consumption of chlorinated pesti-cide residues that are found on food.[3] The problem with using all of this chlorine as a pesticide is that we now know it may be a contributing factor in the development of some of the resistant organ-isms that do not respond to antibiotics.[5,6,7] You may have already heard of these antibiotic-resistant bacteria, or "super bacteria." Exam-ples include certain strains of the MRSA infection and of the *Salmonella* bacteria.[8] These bacteria adapt to the agents that are meant to kill them, and can reproduce and spread disease as a result. They are typi-cally immune to existing medicine, causing panic and placing pressure on scientists and researchers to find a solution quickly.

To reduce your risk of infection from these kinds of bacteria, it is important to reduce your dietary exposure to chlorine compounds, including bleach. This can be done by rinsing all fruits and vegetables (even those already labeled "triple-rinsed") with tap water that you have de-chlorinated using carbon filtration or reverse osmosis. An inexpensive Brita filter can also be used, as it will filter out most chlorine in tap water. It goes without saying that it is important to also avoid consumption of bleached flour and the end products made from bleached flour.

(structures that store bulk material) several times a year to kill grasshopper larvae.[9]

Chlorine solutions are also used post-harvest on fruits, vegetables, eggs, and meat. These and other pesticide applications ensure there will be pesticide exposures occurring every day in the U.S. no matter where we live, what we eat, and what we do for a living.

In Chapter 1, I briefly mentioned that there are allowable mercury levels in the chlorine used to bleach flour.[10] In addition to this mercury, flour may contain pesticide residues.[11,12] According to the USDA Pesticide Data Program (PDP)—a pesticide residue monitoring system—the most common pesticide residues found in wheat and wheat flour are the organophosphate (OP) pesticides known by the names chlorpyrifos, chlorpyrifos methyl, and malathion.[12,13,14] What I mean by "common" is that of the hundreds of wheat samples collected for analysis by the PDP in a given year, up to 66.9 percent of the samples may contain malathion residues and up to 23.1 percent of the samples may contain residues of a chlorpyrifos compound. In some cases, a sample may contain residues of two or more OP pesticide compounds. In the past, these same pesticide residues have also been found in corn.[15,16] Table 3.1, which lists the available PDP data for the most common OP pesticide compounds found in grain samples in recent years, can be found on page 45.[17]

As you can see in Table 3.1, there are some places where data is missing. The USDA PDP did not collect any wheat samples in 2008, 2009, 2010, 2011, 2013, or 2014. In 2012, the USDA collected wheat samples, but did not analyze them for malathion or chlorpyrifos compound residues like they had in 2005 and 2006.[18] In 2009 and 2010, the USDA collected sweet corn samples, but suspiciously found none of the pesticide residues that had been documented in the 2007 and 2008 PDP reports shown in Table 3.1.[19,20]

THE PESTICIDE DATA PROBLEM

According to the Pesticide Data Program's website, the agency "produces the most comprehensive pesticide residue database in the U.S. . . . with an emphasis on those commodities highly consumed by infants and children."[21] However, this is not quite true—the PDP often focuses its

Table 3.1. Common Pesticide Residues Found in Grains Sampled by USDA Pesticide Data Program (PDP)

Grain Commodity —Analysis Year	% of Samples with Chlorpyrifos	% of Samples with Chlorpyrifosmethyl	% of Samples with Malathion
Bleached wheat flour—2004	Not available	20.8% of 151 samples collected	49.4% of 725 samples collected
Wheat—2005	0.6% of 4 samples collected	23.1% of 156 samples collected	66.9% of 451 samples collected
Wheat—2006	0.6% of 4 samples collected	16.7% of 115 samples collected	63% of 433 samples collected
Wheat—2012*	—	—	—
Corn—2007	30% of 195 samples collected	Not available	37.9% of 659 samples collected
Corn—2008	17.8% of 116 samples collected	Not available	33.7% of 219 samples collected

Samples collected but never made public

research on fruits and vegetables, even though grains and wheat are also significant sources of pesticide residue.

Each year, the PDP conducts over 2 million analyses on different fruit, vegetable, and grain crops, but not all commodities are sampled and analyzed every year. Corn samples may be collected one year, and wheat or soybeans the next. Many different fruits and vegetables are collected and analyzed every year for various pesticide residues, but grain samples are not collected and analyzed by the PDP with any regularity. One effect that this has is that people do not generally think about pesticide exposure from eating grains; instead, they have been conditioned to believe that pesticide exposures come primarily from eating fruits and vegetables. Meanwhile, Americans' grain intake is increasing, along with their organophosphate pesticide exposures.

According to a 2016 article published by the prestigious *Journal of the American Medical Association (JAMA)*, from 1999 to 2012, American whole grain intake increased 77 percent, while total fruit and vegetable intake did not change significantly.[22] These findings were derived from data collected by CDC scientists from thousands of Americans through the National Health and Nutrition Examination Survey (NHANES).[22] It is not an easy task to keep track of what and how much Americans eat as time goes on and lifestyles change.

USDA tries to keep track of how much of each commodity Americans eat each year through the food availability per capita data system.[23] (I will provide more details about this in Chapter 4.) In 2013, American corn product consumption was 23.9 pounds per person, while total wheat consumption was 95.1 pounds per person.[23] Wheat consumption data generally includes products such as cereal, pasta, and anything made from wheat flour.[23] Corn products, on the other hand, refer to hominy, grits, corn starch, and any food product made from corn flour or meal.[23] Corn syrup consumption is not part of the corn product tracking system and is instead tracked as part of the sugar consumption data, which I will explain in more detail in Chapter 4.

It is interesting to note that in 2012—when the wheat samples were collected by USDA but *not analyzed* for the most commonly used OP pesticide residues—a major paper was published in the scientific journal *Clinical Epigenetics* on the role of OP pesticide residues in creating conditions for autism development.[24] This paper was published before the 2012 PDP report was made public in February 2014. One can't help but wonder why the USDA did not analyze or report OP pesticide residues on wheat that year, and why the USDA has not conducted any follow-up sampling and analysis of the OP pesticide residues most commonly found on wheat. This follow-up has not been done since 2006, even after wheat samples had been collected in 2012, as Table 3.1 shows.

All of the PDP reports are available on the USDA website for public use.[25] In my opinion, pesticide residue data for *all* grains, including wheat, should be made freely available to the public and easy to access *every* year. It is the public being exposed to pesticides when they eat foods found in the food supply, and American citizens have a right to know the levels of these exposures.

In 2014, the USDA collected and analyzed oat and rice samples— but not wheat—for pesticide residue analyses.[26] It is discouraging that the USDA PDP focused their efforts primarily on these grains, when they are consumed far less frequently than wheat. In 2013, Americans only ate, on average, 3 pounds of oats per person per year and less than 10 pounds of rice per person per year (compared with 95.1 pounds of wheat per year per person, as mentioned on page 46). It would seem more prudent for USDA to collect and analyze *wheat* samples for pesticide residues, since this grain is the most highly consumed and the exposures have been documented in the past. Remember that 67 percent of the 451 wheat samples collected by USDA in 2005 were found to contain the OP pesticide malathion, and nearly 17 percent of 115 wheat samples collected in 2006 contained the OP pesticide chlorpyrifos. When Americans are consuming nearly 100 pounds of wheat per person each year and the USDA is not keeping track of pesticide residues for this grain, how can we ever hope to understand how these exposures add to our body's burden of toxic substances?

HOW PESTICIDES CONTRIBUTE TO DISEASE

You now know that pesticide residue can be found on the foods you eat every day, especially wheat. These pesticides can include substances such as chlorine or the organophosphate pesticides malathion and chlorpyrifos. If these pesticides are used so often in agriculture, however, how can they be harmful to you? The answer lies in the internal damage that even small exposures to pesticides can do over time. Additionally, pesticides can interact with other toxic substances (such as heavy metals) in your body, adding to the strain that is placed on the genes that try to process these heavy loads. The sections below will detail how pesticide exposures can contribute to neurological and metabolic disorders.

Pesticide Co-Exposure

Each pesticide exposure we get from the food we eat is added to our body's existing burden of toxic load and can proceed to interact with other exposures. This is called *co-exposure*. Since the discovery of epigenetics, we cannot say for sure there is a safe exposure level to *any* pesticide because of the numerous possibilities of co-exposure to other toxic substances. Co-exposure may ultimately impact gene function and lead to metabolic impairment and disease.

The OP pesticide residues in the wheat flour used to make bread, cereal, and pasta end up in processed food products.[27,28] One group of scientists found that the flour milling process did not significantly reduce the OP chlorpyrifos pesticides in the wheat, but instead resulted in the distribution of residues in various processed end products.[27] Another group of scientists determined that while losses of pesticide residue do occur during food processing, baking, and boiling, there are still often readily detectable levels of OP pesticide residues in the end products, especially in whole meal or bran-rich breads.[28] So the malathion that is added to the wheat in the grain silos several times a year (see page 43) persists and ends up in the wheat products that you eat.

You may be thinking, "Pesticide exposures must be safe at low levels, or else why would governments allow them?" Maybe these exposures are safe in some cases and under certain circumstances— such as if you are a healthy adult *not* undergoing the aging process or if you are *not* a pregnant woman, developing fetus, child, or adolescent. Co-exposures are becoming a growing cause for concern by public health professionals.

Public Health Professionals Reports

In the case of the chlorpyrifos compounds, the U.S. Public Health Service published a report stating there are concerns about the dietary co-exposure to chlorpyrifos and lead and mercury occurring in pregnant women, infants, and children each and every day.[29] The concerns are related to the neurological impact on child development from co-exposures to these particular substances that are toxic in and of themselves, and potentially far more toxic when they interact with one another in the body.

When you eat the processed foods found in the Western diet, you are being exposed to chlorpyrifos, other OP pesticide compounds, and various heavy metals all at the same time. For example, as you eat a bowl of cereal containing flours made from wheat and corn and the food colors Yellow 5, Red 40, Annatto, Blue 1, and Blue 2, you are potentially being exposed to the heavy metals lead, mercury, and arsenic at the same time as you are being exposed to OP pesticide residues (see Figure 3.1 below). In Chapter 4, we will further discuss all of the heavy metals that are permitted in food colors, preservatives, corn sweeteners, and vegetable oils.

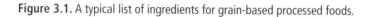

Ingredients: Sugar, corn flour blend (whole grain yellow corn flour, degerminated yellow corn flour), wheat flour, whole grain oat flour, oat fiber, soluble corn fiber, contains 2% of less of partially hydrogenated vegetable oil (coconut, soybean and/or cottonseed), salt, red 40, natural flavor, blue 2, turmeric color, yellow 6, annatto color, blue 1, BHT for freshness.

Vitamins and Minerals: Vitamin C (sodium ascorbate and ascorbic acid), niacinamide, reduced iron, zinc oxide, vitamin B6 (pyridoxine hydrochloride), vitamin B2 (riboflavin), vitamin B1 (thiamin hydrochloride), vitamin A palmitate, folic acid, vitamin D, vitamin B12.

Figure 3.1. A typical list of ingredients for grain-based processed foods.

We do not yet know if these co-exposures are contributing directly to the increasing the number of children with learning disabilities or adults suffering from chronic Western diseases. There are no animal or human studies or data available that examine the toxicity of the interactions among chlorpyrifos, lead, and mercury that are definitely occurring in the human population.[29] There are certainly no models available to determine the cumulative risk of exposure to all of the different toxic substances found in the American diet.

Risk assessment models used in the past to determine the toxicity of exposure to one substance in the workplace cannot easily be adapted to account for *all* of the exposures occurring over a twenty-four-hour period of time from all relevant sources, including diet.[30] Public health professionals are making efforts to address the cumulative risk issue. In 2012, one group of researchers came up with an interesting model to determine the cumulative risk of exposure to OP pesticides for children living in low-income environments.[31] Although the model could incorporate most of the OP pesticide exposures and included parameters to account for changes in dietary intake of protein, fats, and sugars, it did not consider the impact of the dietary co-exposures to the heavy metals lead, mercury, arsenic, and cadmium.[31] The model also did not take into account the role of epigenetics via diet or heavy metal exposure in PON1 gene function.[31]

In 2014, another group of researchers came up with a model to incorporate epigenetic interactions into the risk assessment process for toxic heavy metal exposure.[32] This model, however, did not incorporate the co-exposures to pesticides that are occurring today.[32] The bottom line is there is no official risk assessment process that we can use to determine how *all* of the co-exposures to toxic substances in our diet interact with our genes to promote the development of disease conditions.

What we do know is how *individual* exposures to many of the substances discussed so far can lead to increased risk of disease conditions over time. The following sections will discuss what we know about pesticide exposures with respect to common adult-onset diseases.

Pesticides and Neurological Disease

Millions of people in the U.S. are affected by neurological disorders or diseases.[33] According to the most frequently cited review article on neurological disease occurrence in the U.S. (written by scientists at the Centers for Disease Control and the National Institutes of Health[33]), the two most common late-onset neurological disorders that impact the elderly are Alzheimer's disease and Parkinson's disease.[33] The prevalence for Alzheimer's disease was estimated to be 67 out of 1,000 individuals aged sixty-five or older.[33] The scientists did not include other dementias in their analysis.[33] The prevalence for Parkinson's was estimated to be 9.5 out of 1,000.[33] Autism in children was estimated to be prevalent in just 5.8 out of 1,000 children at the time of the article.[33]

Although the review article was published in 2007, Alzheimer's remains one of the most common neurological diseases in the U.S. In 2013, the Centers for Disease Control (CDC) estimated that there were 5 million Americans afflicted with Alzheimer's.[34] This devastating disease is not part of the normal aging process and is the fifth-leading cause of death among the elderly in the U.S.[34] Death rates for Alzheimer's are increasing, while death rates for heart disease and cancer are decreasing.[34]

Alzheimer's Disease

In a 2013 article, dementia prevalence in the U.S. (including Alzheimer's disease) was reported to be almost 15 percent of the elderly population over the age of seventy years.[35] The cost to society of caring for these dementias during 2010 was estimated to be between $157 billion and $215 billion,[35] with Medicare only covering about $11 billion of the cost.[35] Alzheimer's incidence is increasing across the world, and along with it comes tremendous costs to society.

Figuring out the potential causes of Alzheimer's is key to preventing this condition's occurence. Improvements in diet, the quality of the food supply, and health education could lead to significant reductions in the number of afflicted people and the costs associated with caring for them. The role of diet in the development of Alzheimer's is clear.[36] Intake of saturated and trans fats, low levels of vitamin D, and low levels of methyl-donating nutrients are all associated with significant increased risk of developing Alzheimer's.[36] Health education could address these dietary issues, as well as some of the lifestyle factors—such as inadequate exercise and smoking—that are known to increase risk of Alzheimer's.[36]

Many risk factors are directly or indirectly related to the gene-environment interactions that likely cause Alzheimer's disease.[36] Pesticide exposures (specifically exposures to organophosphate pesticides) are independently associated with Alzheimer's and dementia, even without considering dietary co-exposures to other toxic substances and many of the other risk factors.

The most powerful and impressive study to date that links pesticide exposure with the development of dementia and Alzheimer's was published in 2010.[37] Researchers in Utah followed 3,084 residents living in an agricultural community over a ten-year period to see if any would develop dementia or Alzheimer's disease.[37] Of the residents enrolled in the study, 572 participants reported using pesticides as part of their agricultural work.[37] At the beginning of the study, each participant was sixty-five years of age or older and free of any dementia.[37] Cognitive assessments were done at the beginning of the study and after three, seven, and ten years.[37] Five hundred of the individuals enrolled in the study developed dementia over time, and of those, 344 had a secondary diagnosis of Alzheimer's disease.[37]

The researchers analyzed their data after adjusting for age at the beginning of the study, gender, and level of education. Additionally, they considered each participant's APOE gene status.[37] APOE gene variation is associated with Alzheimer's; if you happen to carry a variation of the APOE gene (APOE-e4) you will have a higher risk of developing Alzheimer's.[38] If you drink alcohol and have the APOE-e4 gene variation, then you are at significant risk of developing Alzheimer's disease.[39] After making all of these risk factors equal (adjusting), the researchers in Utah found that occupational exposure to organophosphate pesticides was linked to a significantly higher risk of developing Alzheimer's disease.[37] When exposures to different pesticides (carbamates, DDT, and methyl bromides) were analyzed, the risk of Alzheimer's was still higher in the organophosphate pesticide exposure group.[37]

The Utah study was powerful both because of the sheer number of participants in the study and the fact that 90 percent of them were members of the Church of Jesus Christ of Latter Day Saints (also known as Mormons).[37] As a rule, Mormons do not smoke tobacco or drink alcohol and caffeinated beverages. For these reasons, they generally tend to be healthier. The characteristics of the residents of the Utah community meant that some of the risk factors normally associated with Alzheimer's were not in play, making this study tightly controlled.

It is important to note that one weakness of the Utah study was that the researchers did not consider the *dietary* pesticide exposures—the study's focus was on *occupational* exposure. The study also did not consider co-exposures to other toxic substances in the food supply, which may have played a factor in the development of Alzheimer's. Fortunately, there are a couple of great, more recent review articles that discuss the cumulative risk of neurological disease associated with organophosphate pesticide exposures when there are co-exposures to heavy metals.[40, 41]

For example, a 2015 article reviewed the collective effects of toxic metals, pesticides, industrial and commercial pollutants, antimicrobials (often the active ingredients of soaps and toothpastes), and air pollutants. Although the researchers concluded that more extensive studies are needed to determine the risk that co-exposures to these substances pose, they noted that most of the agents they reviewed disrupt the endocrine system and can impair brain function. With all of these environmental substances combined, the number of people who are diagnosed with Alzheimer's is bound to increase in the coming years.[40]

Another article published in 2015 looked at how environmental factors affected the brain mechanisms that can cause both Alzheimer's and Parkinson's disease. For example, the authors noted that the metals arsenic, lead, and cadmium (which we have discussed in Chapter 1) together produced a "synergic effect" in the brain—a sharp increase in proteins and enzymes that form plaques found in the brains of Alzheimer's disease patients.

As for Parkinson's disease, the researchers stated that 90 percent of Parkinson's cases cannot be solely attributed to hereditary factors, suggesting that there are multiple environmental factors that contribute to this condition. Dozens of the reviewed studies demonstrated a significantly higher incidence of Parkinson's disease in subjects who were exposed to professional-use pesticides than in unexposed subjects. This study concluded with a note that environmental exposures to metals, pesticides, and other toxic substances can alter a person's genes, and that even early or fetal exposures can contribute to Alzheimer's or Parkinson's disease development down the line.[41]

Parkinson's Disease

Parkinson's disease is a relatively common neurological disease that is often characterized by irregularities in the motor system, such as trembling, stiffness, and difficulty standing or walking. Since Parkinson's disease affects so many people—about 500,000 people are affected, and many more are undiagnosed—and has no known cure, it is important to understand the potential risk factors.[42]

One risk factor for developing Parkinson's is exposure to organophosphate pesticides.[41] One recent study, conducted by researchers at the University of California Los Angeles (UCLA) campus, provided strong evidence that household organophosphate pesticide use is associated with the development of Parkinson's disease.[43] As I mentioned earlier in this chapter, two of the OP pesticides most commonly found in wheat are malathion and chlorpyrifos. These pesticides can also be found in products used for killing insects or other pests in the household.

The UCLA researchers studied 357 individuals with Parkinson's disease (who had their diagnosis for at least three years) and 807 individuals who did not have Parkinson's. The subjects' household use of malathion, chlorpyrifos, and other organophosphate pesticides was examined.[43] Household use of pesticides was characterized by the residents' frequency of using specific products—such as liquids, granules, and baits and powders—to kill ants, cockroaches, termites, flies, weeds, spiders, termites, and hornets.[43] After controlling for other variables known to contribute to the risk of developing Parkinson's, the researchers found that the frequent use of pesticides containing general OP compounds increased the odds of getting Parkinson's disease by 71 percent.[43] Using the OP compounds in the class to which malathion and chlorpyrifos belong doubled the odds of developing Parkinson's.[43]

The UCLA study is even more interesting from the PON1 gene standpoint. As you may recall from Chapter 2, the PON1 gene helps to break down OP pesticides in the body. However, certain PON1 variants are known to be slow metabolizers of these pesticides. The researchers determined the PON1 gene variation in 73 percent of the participants.[43] They found that the participants who were carriers of the "slow" PON1 variants were at significantly higher risk of developing Parkinson's when using household pesticides containing OP.[43] This finding is the first of its kind to show the importance of limiting exposures to organophosphate pesticides to prevent neurological disease. The researchers did not consider or incorporate the analysis of dietary factors or co-exposures to heavy metals in their study.

Neurological disorders are not the only conditions to which pesticide exposures can contribute. In the next section, we will discuss the role of organophosphate pesticide exposures in metabolic diseases, such as heart disease, cancer, and type 2 diabetes.

Pesticides and Metabolic Diseases

A *metabolic disease* is a condition that is caused by abnormal chemical reactions and negatively affects the cell's ability to perform important actions, such as breaking down food into its different components.[44] Diabetes is one of the most well-known metabolic diseases, and emerging evidence suggests cancer is primarily a metabolic disease as well.[45,46] Having a group of metabolic conditions is a risk factor for heart disease. Heart disease and cancer are the top two causes of death in the elderly and middle-aged populations across most ethnic groups.[47]

Patients with type 2 diabetes have an increased risk of developing cancers.[46] This is because humans with type 2 diabetes have high levels of glucose, and these levels contribute to tumor growth.[46] The elevated glucose levels feed the cancer cells. Elevated glucose levels and type 2 diabetes also increase your risk of heart disease and stroke[48] and your risk of dying from a sudden heart attack.[49] Fifty percent of heart attack deaths occur in people with heart disease and of those, about half were never previously diagnosed with heart disease.[49] The glucose levels in your blood are a key indicator of your metabolic health and your risk of heart disease and cancer. Glucose levels can be controlled with proper diet and adequate exercise. As part of a proper diet, I recommend eating foods that are free of organophosphate pesticide residues. I will tell you how to find such foods in Chapter 8.

There is strong evidence to support the theory that consuming wheat with malathion and chlorpyrifos pesticide residues will lead to elevated glucose levels. In two studies, rats fed malathion and low levels of chlorpyrifos showed increased glucose levels within twenty-eight days.[50,51] The researchers concluded that exposures to these organophosphate pesticides may increase the risk of diabetes in humans.[50,51] In a human study conducted by researchers in Iraq, non-diabetic farmers exposed to malathion over fifteen to twenty years showed increasing levels of malathion in their blood.[52] The higher the malathion levels became, the more likely the farmers were to develop diabetes.[52]

There is a need for more research in the U.S. on this correlation between grain consumption and heart disease, diabetes, and cancer. Ideally, a study would be conducted to determine if there is a *direct* link between the dietary intake of OP-contaminated wheat products by Americans and their glucose levels, leading to an increased risk of developing diabetes. The Centers for Disease Control and Prevention (CDC) has the data available to look for these links, but incredibly, no studies have been funded by the U.S. government as of 2016.

Each year, the CDC keeps track of American dietary intake and correlates it with toxic substance exposure data through the National Health and Nutrition Examination Survey (NHANES).[53] The NHANES dataset includes this dietary survey information and the corresponding blood and urine levels for a variety of heavy metals and pesticides, including malathion and chlorpyrifos.[53] This dataset has been used by several research teams to find a link between organophosphate pesticide exposures and autism and ADHD. In Chapter 6, I will discuss these findings and the role of pesticide exposures in causing these debilitating childhood diseases in more detail.

In the meantime, I recommend eating an organic diet to reduce your organophosphate pesticide exposures and prevent the development of diabetes and other metabolic conditions. If you begin to use organic wheat flour, be sure to store it in a sealed plastic bag in the refrigerator, or it will get moldy due to the lack of chlorine and may also become infested with insects due to the lack of pesticide residues. Putting the flour in the fridge is a small price to pay to ensure your diet is clear of these residues! See Chapter 8 for more ways to create a safe food supply in your home.

CONCLUSION

After reading this chapter, it should be clear to you by now that the organophosphate pesticide exposures from the food you eat (especially wheat) can contribute to the development of numerous neurological and metabolic disease conditions. Your ability to maintain good health will depend largely on the quality of the food you eat, whether it is pesticide-free or not, and your body's ability to rid itself of the organophosphate pesticide residues that will no doubt make their way into your body when you eat processed foods. Co-exposures to other toxic substances, such as heavy metals, suppress the PON1 gene activity needed to break down these substances. The consumption of these substances needs to be reduced whenever possible to optimize your health. In the next chapter, you will learn how to reduce your intake of food ingredients at risk for heavy metal contamination.

4.

Ingredients That Add Heavy Metals to Your Body

In the previous chapter, I discussed how food—especially grains and wheat—can have pesticide residues, exposing you to substances that can cause a number of conditions. In this chapter, we will focus on how some other common food ingredients may contribute to the development of disease by depositing toxic heavy metals into our bodies. Vegetable oils, food colors, corn syrups, and preservatives are examples of these ingredients—found mostly in processed food products—that will contribute to your body's burden of heavy metal exposure. Although few studies have been conducted to determine the concentrations of heavy metals in food products, there seems to be some evidence to suggest the most common toxic heavy metals found in the food supply are inorganic mercury, lead, cadmium, and arsenic.[1,2,3,4]

Scientists have determined that the concentrations of heavy metals in foods eaten by adults and children correlate with the heavy metals found in their bloodstream.[5] This is an important finding because some Western diseases are associated with elevated levels of lead, mercury, cadmium, or arsenic in the bloodstream.[6,7,8] The greater the dietary exposure to these heavy metals, the more elevated they become in the bloodstream. Elevated levels of lead, arsenic, cadmium, and/or mercury in the bloodstream have been found to increase the risk of developing obesity, diabetes, and/or heart disease.[6,7,8] To reduce your risk of developing these chronic diseases, you will want to avoid food ingredients allowed to contain these heavy metal impurities. We will start with the food ingredients that Americans eat the most of and go from there.

VEGETABLE OILS AND INORGANIC MERCURY

As was mentioned in Chapter 1, the average American consumes 36 pounds of vegetable oils per year. Vegetable oils include coconut oil, canola oil, soybean oil, olive oil, sunflower oil, and palm oil, among other varieties. Many of these oils are processed with mercury cell chlor-alkali chemicals and therefore may contain trace amounts of mercury. We know this because a crucial report was published in 2013 as a reference document by FEDIOL, the trade organization for members of the European Union (EU) vegetable oil and protein meal industry.[9] FEDIOL conducted a risk assessment of the chain of vegetable oil products manufactured using the common *alkali* refining process and found a moderate risk of mercury contamination.

During this refining process, a chlor-alkali product called sodium hydroxide (also known as caustic soda) is added to the older, degraded vegetable oils to remove free fatty acids.[9] These acids must be removed to enhance the value and taste[9] of the oils; otherwise, there would be a bitter or rancid flavor in the food products containing these vegetable oils.[9] Table 4.1 below provides a list of the vegetable oils at risk of mercury contamination due to this alkali refining process[9,10,11] and their common uses in food products.

Table 4.1. Vegetable Oils at Moderate Risk of Mercury Contamination and Food Products Potentially Impacted

Vegetable Oil Type	Common Uses in Food Products
Coconut oil	Baked goods, pastries
Olive oil	Salad dressings
Palm oil	Almond butter, cookies
Rapeseed (canola) oil	Chips, crackers, frozen fish sticks, frozen French fries, mayonnaise, peanut butter, salad dressings
Soybean oil	Bread, cookies, crackers, frozen fish sticks, frozen French fries, frozen TV dinners, horseradish, mayonnaise, peanut butter, salad dressings, tartar sauce
Sunflower oil	Chips, crackers, frozen French fries

Americans have increased their consumption of vegetable oils significantly since 1970. Overconsumption of these oils not only likely contributes to your mercury exposure, but also promotes the development of heart disease and diabetes.[12] Table 4.2 below shows the changes in vegetable oil and fat consumption over the last forty years in the U.S. The data was extracted from the United States Department of Agriculture (USDA) food availability system and has been adjusted for loss or spoilage so it more nearly reflects actual consumption.[13]

Table 4.2. Refined Vegetable Oil and Fat Consumption in the United States

Commodity	1970 per capita consumption (lbs/year)	2010 per capita consumption (lbs/year)	Percent increase or decrease (rounded)
Butter	3.3	3.4	+3%
Cooking oil (including canola, cottonseed, peanut, soybean, sunflower seed, vegetable)	10.3	36.0	+250%
Margarine	6.6	2.1	−68%
Shortening	8.9	7.9	−11%
TOTAL	29.1	49.4	+70%

Table 4.2 shows that in 1970, the average American ate 29.1 pounds per year of refined vegetable oils and fats. By 2010, this number had increased by 70 percent to 49.4 pounds of oils and fats consumed per person per year. During the 1970–2010 time period, shortening and margarine consumption decreased by 11 percent and 68 percent respectively, while butter consumption increased by a mere 3 percent. On the other hand, consumption of refined vegetable oil—the most chemically processed ingredient out of these four substances—increased by 250 percent, accounting for nearly the entire increase in general fats consumption.

In Chapter 5, we will discuss how this drastic change in American refined vegetable oil consumption has contributed to the development of ADHD, autism, and other chronic Western disease conditions. Until then, it is important for you to note that the manufacturing process of vegetable oils involves the extensive use of at least two chlor-alkali chemicals[14,15,16] that may be a source of dietary inorganic mercury exposure,[9] and this exposure may impact gene function.[17,18] Another common ingredient that may be a source of mercury exposure is corn sweetener. However, in the case of this ingredient, mercury is purposely added during the manufacturing process.

CORN SWEETENERS AND INORGANIC MERCURY

Corn sweeteners are made from corn starch, the same material manufactured over 150 years ago for the laundry business.[19] Corn starch is made from corn using the wet milling manufacturing process, which separates the corn kernel into starch, gluten, germ, and fiber.[19] The

---

The Corn Sweetener Manufacturing Process

Corn, as you typically picture it, is on the cob or in a can. How does this food become a sweetener, added to foods that taste nothing like corn? As you read above, the wet milling manufacturing process separates the corn kernel into four parts: The starch, gluten, germ, and fiber. While the gluten, germ, and fiber are further processed into feed for animals, the starch is washed and refined into corn sweeteners and ethanol.[19]

As part of the washing process, the starch is softened as it is cleaned (steeped in sulfur dioxide or a slightly acidic sulfurous acid solution[20]). Next, *mercuric chloride* is added to the mix to inhibit naturally occurring starch-degrading enzymes that are produced by bacteria.[20] The resulting steep liquor is discarded, as the corn starch mixture is strained over and over again with water to remove any remaining fiber, germ, or gluten.[20] Finally, the starch is dried; this is the material from which corn sweeteners are made.

starch is the part that is used for corn sweeteners. During the process that turns it into sweetener, a mercury compound called *mercuric chloride* is added to prevent starch-degrading enzymes from occurring. (See "The Corn Sweetener Manufacturing Process" inset on page 62 for more details on the wet milling manufacturing process.)

There are several different corn sweeteners made from corn starch, with the most refined product being *high fructose corn syrup* (HFCS). For this reason, HFCS is viewed as the "end product" of the corn wet milling process. Table 4.3 lists the most common corn sweeteners found in the Western diet, including HFCS, and the food products in which they are most frequently found:

Table 4.3. Corn Sweeteners at Risk of Mercury Contamination and Food Products Potentially Impacted

Corn sweetener	Common uses in food products
Corn syrup	Candy, caramel topping, chocolate syrup, Japanese-style noodle soup, ketchup, lunch meat, TV dinners
Dextrose	Assorted cookies and crackers, candy, cereal, hot dogs, pancake mix, sausage, toaster pastries, TV dinners
High fructose corn syrup	Canned spaghetti and soups, caramel topping, chocolate syrup, ketchup, pancake syrup, pork and beans, salad dressings, soft drinks, teriyaki marinade, toaster pastries
Maltodextrin	Assorted chips,crackers, Japanese-style noodle soup, stuffing mix
Modified corn starch	Cake mix, pancake mix, TV dinners

Inorganic Mercury Exposure from Corn Sweeteners

Any of the corn sweeteners listed in Table 4.3 have the potential to contain mercury. During the corn sweetener refining process, several chemicals are added to the mix, including sodium hydroxide (caustic soda), hydrogen chloride, alpha-amylase, gluco-amylase, isomerase, filter aid, powdered carbon, calcium chloride, and magnesium sulfate.[21] As was previously mentioned in Chapter 1, sodium hydroxide and hydrogen chloride are used routinely to regulate the acidity (pH) of food products during manufacturing processes. These same chemicals are used in the corn sweetener refining process and may contain mercury residues.

Because current international food standards allow one microgram (µg) of mercury in each gram (g) of caustic soda (or 1 ppm),[22,23] there is a chance mercury exposure may occur from the consumption of corn sweeteners due to their manufacturing processes. Studies have been published that report the amount of mercury residue found in HFCS or food products containing HFCS or corn syrup.[1,24,25] For example, one study found mercury in 45 percent of the HFCS samples that the researchers tested. Of these mercury-containing samples, the level of mercury content ranged from 0.012 micrograms of mercury per gram of HFCS to 0.570 µg/g.[1] It is unclear whether the mercury residue in these samples was from the use of the mercury cell chemicals or the mercuric chloride that was added purposely to the corn starch at the beginning of the refinery process.

It is probably safe to assume that if you eat any products containing the corn sweeteners listed in Table 4.3 on page 63, there is an excellent chance you will be exposed to mercury. In 2013, my collaborators and I conducted a study at a community college in which students were asked to eliminate corn sweeteners from their diet. We collected blood samples at the end of the intervention; the one student who was unable to eliminate corn sweeteners from her diet had the highest inorganic mercury levels of all.[26] Her mercury level was 5.01 nanograms per gram, compared with 1.325 ng/g, which was the average mercury level of the group of participants who eliminated corn sweeteners from their diets. In Chapter 5, I will talk more about our findings from this study.

There is no doubt in my mind that corn sweetener consumption may be a source of inorganic mercury exposure. Along with the consumption of other mercury-containing ingredients in processed foods, corn sweetener also may contribute to the rising incidences of Western diseases, such as heart disease and diabetes. In the next section, you will see just how large a spike corn sweetener consumption experienced between 1970 and 2014.

History of Corn Syrup Consumption in the U.S.

In 1970, the average American ate 69.1 pounds per year of refined sugar. The type of sugar consumed was primarily cane and beet sugar. With the introduction of the new processing technology for making HFCS in the mid-1980s, sugar use switched from cane and beet sugar to HFCS, which was less expensive. Food manufacturers began adding HFCS, instead of sugar derived from sugar cane and beets, to beverages and other processed foods. Table 4.4 below shows the changes in refined sugar consumption over forty-four years in the U.S. The data was extracted from the USDA food availability system and is adjusted for loss or spoilage so that it more nearly reflects actual consumption.[13]

Table 4.4. Refined Sugar Consumption in the United States

Commodity	1970 per capita consumption (lbs/year)	2014 per capita consumption (lbs/year)	Percent increase or decrease (rounded)
Cane and beet sugar	59.8	40.1	−32.9%
Total corn sweeteners (excluding high fructose corn syrup)	9.0	8.8	-2.2%
High fructose corn syrup	0.3	26.8	+8833%
TOTAL refined sugar	69.1	75.7	+9.5%

As you can see from Table 4.4, the average American consumed 75.7 pounds per year of refined sugar in 2014, increasing their overall intake of refined sugar by 9.5 percent compared to 1970. This increase in overall refined sugar consumption does not seem very large, but when you look at the changes in the *type* of sugar being consumed, it becomes clear there has been a tremendous change in corn sweetener consumption from 1970 to 2014. Per capita consumption of HFCS increased 8833 percent from 1970 to 2014.

In Chapter 5, we will discuss how this immense change in HFCS consumption has contributed to the development of neurological disorders and other chronic disease conditions. In the meantime, remember that consumption of HFCS in processed food is reported to be a source of dietary inorganic mercury exposure,[1,24,25] and this exposure may impact gene function.[17,26] It is also important to note that refined sugars, including HFCS, do not contain any vitamins or minerals. Their consumption may actually lead to reductions in the dietary intake of life-sustaining vitamins and minerals.[27]

FOOD COLORS AND HEAVY METALS

From time to time, you may notice in your supermarket foods such as gelatin, syrups, candy, cereals, sports drinks, and canned fruits in a variety of bright or unusual hues. Although these foods grab your attention, they often are eaten at a price.

Food colors that are made from chemicals derived from sodium hydroxide and petroleum may contain allowable levels of mercury and other heavy metals. Petroleum comes from the ground, where heavy metals are also found. These food colors are expected to contain trace amounts of the heavy metals mercury, lead, and/or arsenic as a result of their extraction and manufacturing processes.[28] In the U.S., the Food and Drug Administration (FDA) requires that these synthetic food colors be tested and certified to ensure they only contain up to the allowable levels of mercury, lead, or arsenic.[28] Food colors derived from plants or minerals do not undergo this certification process (see "Other Food Colors of Concern" on page 69).

In the European Union (EU) and the United Kingdom (UK), however, food products containing some of these colors must carry a mandatory warning on the label: *"May have an adverse effect on activity and attention in children."*[29,30] The only difference between the food colors used in the U.S. and Europe is the identification numbers used by the food manufacturers. For example, on food products produced in the U.S., Sunset Yellow is denoted as "Yellow 6" on the food ingredient label. But if the product is sold in the EU, Sunset Yellow is denoted as "E-110," and the food package must carry the mandatory warning to parents.

Table 4.5 on page 67 shows the FDA-certified allowable amounts of heavy metal impurities in common food colors. Some colors are known by more than one name. The table also names food products in which these colors are commonly found as ingredients. Note the food colors with an asterisk (*) beside them. These colors must carry the mandatory warning label if they are sold in the EU or United Kingdom.[29,30] This warning label requirement was a direct outcome of research conducted by scientists in Europe (see "European Food Color Research" below).

Table 4.5. Specifications for Common Food Colors in the United States Requiring Certification by FDA

Color Names	Allowable Impurities	Common Uses
Blue 1	Arsenic ≤ 3 ppm Chromium ≤ 50 ppm Lead ≤ 10 ppm	Candy, cheese flavored snacks, chocolate and strawberry syrups, colored ice cream cones, power drinks, soft drinks, spicy corn chips, sugar sweetened cereals
Blue 2	Arsenic ≤ 3 ppm Lead ≤ 10 ppm Mercury ≤ 1 ppm	Candy, energy drinks
Yellow 5 / E-102* / Tartrazine	Arsenic ≤ 3 ppm Lead ≤ 10 ppm Mercury ≤ 1 ppm	Barbeque flavored snacks, boxed macaroni and cheese, butter, cheese, cheese flavored snacks, ice cream, soft drinks, spicy corn chips, sweet pickle relish, vitamin water
Yellow 6 / E-110* / Sunset Yellow	Arsenic ≤ 3 ppm Lead ≤ 10 ppm Mercury ≤ 1 ppm	Cheese flavored snacks, chocolate syrup, ice cream, power drinks, pudding snacks, sugar sweetened cereals, sugarless gum
Red 40 / E-129* / Allura Red	Arsenic ≤ 3 ppm Lead ≤ 10 ppm	Canned cherries, cherry pie filling, children's cough medicine, cotton candy, energy drinks, gelatin mix and snack, ice cream, liquid aspirin, soft drinks, strawberry cake mix, sugar sweetened cereals, vitamin water

≤ means less than or equal to

European Food Color Research

In Europe, several human studies have been conducted by researchers. These studies show that consumption of Yellow 5 and/or Yellow 6 negatively impacts child health.[31,32] Dr. Neil Ward determined the effects of Yellow 5 and Yellow 6 on children with and without hyperactivity.[31,32] He found that only hyperactive children showed significant losses in zinc (a nutrient needed to build heavy metal-eliminating MT proteins in the body) after drinking beverages containing Yellow 5 and Yellow 6.[31,32] The children who were not hyperactive showed no changes in their zinc status after consuming the same beverages.[31,32] What this means is that there is something in these yellow food colors that creates conditions for zinc loss in children with ADHD. I believe it is the allowable heavy metal impurities.

The connection between the dietary intake of food colors and hyperactivity in children continues to be studied by researchers in Europe. While Dr. Ward[31,32] studied the metabolic impact of zinc loss in hyperactive children who consumed food colors Yellow 5 and Yellow 6, other researchers have focused their studies on the impact of food color consumption on the behavior of children in the general population. In the UK, researchers found a negative effect on the behavior of 1,873 three-year-olds when parents reported their children became hyperactive after consuming a drink containing a mixture of food colors and sodium benzoate, a food additive that is used as a preservative.[33] It was unclear, however, whether the food colors or the sodium benzoate caused the hyperactivity in the children.[33] (See page 73 for more information on sodium benzoate.)

To clarify the findings, a new study was commissioned by the UK government. The research was led by a different group of scientists and the results were published in 2007.[34] This time, both three-year-old and eight-year-old children from the general population were included in the study.[34] The children were divided into three groups and given different beverages to drink; one group consumed a beverage mixed with sodium benzoate alone, another group consumed a beverage with food colorings alone, and the remaining group consumed a placebo beverage with no exposure to either sodium benzoate or food colors.[34]

The results of this new study confirmed that the consumption of beverages containing food colors or sodium benzoate by children in both age groups resulted in increased hyperactivity.[34] Both parents and teachers reported observing the increased hyperactivity in the children who drank the beverages containing food colors or sodium benzoate.[34] The study included children in the general population, not just hyperactive children, and the results made it clear that the dietary intake of food colorings or sodium benzoate may affect the behavior of all children.[34] It was this study that led to the requirement in the EU and the UK that food products containing certain food colors must carry the mandatory warning on their labels, *"May have an adverse effect on activity and attention in children."*[29,30] The U.S. does not yet require such a warning. This may be because no similar studies on the effects of food colors in children have been funded or researched by the U.S. government as of 2016, as I will discuss in the next section.

U.S. Food Color Research

To my knowledge, there has been no research funded by the U.S. government to determine the impact of food color consumption on child health. However, unfunded research does occur. In 2009, my collaborators and I followed up on Dr. Ward's work and published a peer-reviewed model explaining how zinc losses may occur from the consumption of food colors containing allowable levels of mercury.[2] We explained how these losses may impact MT gene function, weakening the child's immune system and ability to learn.[2] Mercury and other heavy metals in food colors may displace zinc from the binding sites on the metal transporter protein, metallothionein (MT), which is produced by the MT gene (refer back to Chapter 2 for more information about the MT gene).[2] The end result of this zinc displacement may be an overall loss of zinc from the body via urinary excretion. The more heavy metal exposure a child has, the more likely he will become zinc deficient as the zinc is released from his body.[2,35]

Other Food Colors of Concern

In addition to the FDA-certified food colors, there are some other food color ingredients on the market that may contain allowable levels of the heavy metals arsenic, lead, and mercury. These colors are exempt from FDA analysis and certification because they are not made from petroleum; they are instead derived from plants or minerals[36] found in the natural environment. Beware of buying food products that claim they are made from "natural" ingredients, however. These products may contain naturally-derived food colors that will contribute to your heavy metal burden. These food color ingredients are not "safer" for you to consume.[37] Table 4.6 below provides information found in the United States Code of Federal Regulations about these FDA-exempt food colors and their allowable impurity levels.[38]

Table 4.6. Specifications for Less Common Food Colors in the United States—Exempt from Certification Requirements

Color names, synonyms	Allowable impurities	Common Uses
Annatto	Arsenic ≤ 3 ppm Lead ≤ 10 ppm	Buttery spread, cheddar cheese, cheese spread, ice cream, sugar sweetened cereal,
Beta carotene	Arsenic ≤ 3 ppm Lead ≤ 10 ppm	Canned tropical fruit, fat-free and cholesterol-free liquid egg product, vegetable oil spread
Caramel	Arsenic ≤ 3 ppm Lead ≤ 10 ppm Mercury ≤ 0.1 ppm	Beef gravy, candy, canned peppers, chocolate syrup, ice cream, lunch meat, pancake syrup, soft drinks, spice rub
Carmine, cochineal extract	Arsenic ≤ 3 ppm Lead ≤ 10 ppm	Canned fruit cocktail
Spirulina	Arsenic ≤ 2 ppm Lead ≤ 2 ppm Mercury ≤ 1 ppm	Health food products
Titanium dioxide	Arsenic ≤ 1 ppm Lead ≤ 10 ppm Mercury ≤ 1 ppm	Vitamins and supplements

≤ *means less than or equal to*

It is a shame that spirulina may contain these harmful heavy metals, because it is considered a "superfood"[39] that provides vitamins and minerals needed for proper gene function. In a recent study, researchers verified the consistent finding of mercury in twenty-five different products containing the spirulina ingredient.[40]

PRESERVATIVES CONTAINING LEAD

In addition to the vegetable oils, corn sweeteners, and food colors discussed in this chapter, there are also many food ingredient chemicals that are allowed to contain small amounts of heavy metals.[41] These chemicals are used as preservatives in the food supply. Preservatives are added to food to slow spoilage, prevent foodborne illness-causing bacteria, and enhance the taste or appearance of food, according to the FDA website.[42]

However, these benefits are outweighed by the possibility of severe disease conditions that can occur as a result of the heavy metals allowed in these preservatives. Lead is the most commonly found heavy metal allowed in these food ingredients. You may remember from Chapter 2 that lead is not safe to consume at *any* level and is a factor in the development of Alzheimer's disease, ADHD, and pervasive developmental delay, especially when the diet is deficient in calcium.[43,44,45,46] Lead exposure can and does interfere with memory and the learning process. Therefore, you may want to reduce or avoid consumption of the food ingredients listed in Table 4.7 below that are allowed to contain small amounts of lead.[41,47,48,49,50]

Table 4.7. Limits for Heavy Metals in Food Additives Used as Preservatives

Preservative Name	Allowable Impurities	Common Uses
Calcium chloride	Lead ≤ 2 ppm	Canned vegetables, dill relish, frozen TV dinners, organic frozen pizza, power drinks, sweet pickle relish, sweet pickles
Carrageenan	Arsenic ≤ 3 ppm Cadmium ≤ 2 ppm Lead ≤ 5 ppm Mercury ≤ 1 ppm	Almond milk, canned evaporated milk, cottage cheese, ice cream, organic soy milk, pudding mix, sour cream
Citric acid	Lead ≤ 0.5 ppm	Barbeque sauce, energy drinks, organic strawberry preserves, organic tomato sauce, powdered spice mix

≤ means less than or equal to

Monosodium L-Glutamate, sodium glutamate, MSG	Lead ≤ 1 ppm	Hot dogs, sausage
Potassium chloride	Lead ≤ 2 ppm	Canned ham, frozen TV dinners
Sodium benzoate	Lead ≤ 2 ppm Mercury ≤ 1 ppm	Ginger ale, lunch meat, salad dressing, soft drinks, soy sauce, tonic water
Sodium diacetate	Lead ≤ 2 ppm	Lunch meat, hot dogs
Sodium nitrite	Lead ≤ 2 ppm	Bacon, beef jerky, canned ham, hot dogs, lunch meat, sausage

≤ means less than or equal to

Notice that sodium benzoate is one of the preservatives with allowable impurities of lead and inorganic mercury. Earlier in this chapter, we discussed the role of sodium benzoate in creating hyperactivity in children and the studies that were conducted in Europe to draw this conclusion.[33,34] Dietary co-exposures to lead and inorganic mercury from foods containing sodium benzoate could be contributing factors in creating hyperactivity. (See inset "Spotlight on Sodium Benzoate" on page 73.)

FDA HEAVY METAL MONITORING PROGRAM

After reading about all of the heavy metals allowed in food ingredients, you are probably wondering if the FDA has some kind of program in place to monitor the amount of heavy metals actually found in the American food supply. FDA does indeed have a monitoring program, called the "Total Diet Study." The purpose of the program is to monitor America's intake of foodborne contaminants.[55] Four times a year, FDA workers go shopping at the same grocery stores that you do and buy about 280 different foods during a *market basket survey*.[55] The regulatory agency then prepares these foods as you would and analyzes them for various chemical contaminants, including pesticides, heavy metals, and radioactive materials.[55] Examples

Spotlight on Sodium Benzoate

Sodium benzoate is not found naturally in the environment.[50] The food ingredient is manufactured three different ways. One of these methods involves using sodium hydroxide (which may contain mercury residue[22,23,51]) in the neutralization of benzoic acid.[50] Sodium benzoate is the end product of this neutralization. The chemical is used as a food additive (preservative) to control microbial, or bacterial, growth, and as a flavoring agent. It is most commonly found in soft drinks and cough syrup. In soft drinks, the chemical can combine with ascorbic acid (vitamin C) to form benzene, a chemical compound that may cause cancer. When used as a preservative, sodium benzoate must not legally contain more than the allowable level of 2 ppm lead.[52,53] Manufacturing product specification sheets indicate food-grade sodium benzoate may contain up to 1 ppm mercury.[54]

of foods that are analyzed by the FDA during its market basket survey include baby food, infant formula, chocolate syrup, grains, meats, assorted vegetables, and fruits.[56] The more processed the foods, the more likely it is contaminants will be found.[56]

Whether or not contaminants are found depends on the analytical method used to measure the heavy metal being studied. In the case of mercury, the monitoring results for the years 2008 and 2009 were omitted by FDA due to "issues in methodology."[56] The food samples collected by the total diet study during the years 2010 and 2011 were not analyzed for mercury.[56] Some food samples collected after 2011 have been analyzed for mercury, but the new methodology is not stated in the updated FDA report.[56] According to the 2016 publication, FDA reports finding mercury only in products containing fish.[56] Since the methodology is not known and mercury was found only in products containing fish, we must assume the new methodology focuses exclusively on detecting the organic form of mercury.

It is interesting to note that in 2009, two studies published by two different research groups determined there were detectable levels of mercury in a variety of foods found in American grocery stores.[1,25] My collaborators and I published our findings of mercury in high fructose corn syrup in the first paper.[1] In the second paper, researchers at the Institute for Agriculture and Trade Policy reported finding mercury in foods containing high fructose corn syrup.[25] Canadian researchers duplicated our findings in 2010.[24] Since these publications, the FDA has experienced difficulty with their mercury monitoring program and reports finding mercury only in fish and food products containing fish.[56] There is obviously a significant difference between the findings of third-party researchers and the FDA when mercury levels are being investigated in the food supply.

Why would FDA only look for organic mercury and not inorganic mercury, when the evidence suggests inorganic mercury is a widespread contaminant in the food supply? Organic methylmercury in fish is a known and accepted contaminant. Mercury exposure from fish consumption is an easy problem to address. FDA simply advises consumers to limit their fish intake to reduce their mercury exposures.[57] In this book, we have been focusing on the *inorganic* mercury in the food supply—a controversial contaminant because it is widespread and permeates the processed food supply. I cannot imagine the FDA advising consumers to avoid eating processed foods.

Inorganic mercury in the food supply is an inconvenient truth. Fixing exposure to inorganic mercury is harder than simply reducing your intake of certain foods. However, reducing our exposure is extremely important: The American Academy of Pediatrics published a technical report on mercury in the environment in 2001 which concluded, "Mercury in all of its forms is toxic to the fetus and children, and efforts should be made to reduce exposure to the extent possible to pregnant women and children as well as the general population."[58] Information about inorganic mercury sources and their effects must be more accessible to the public. The FDA should educate consumers on the potential consequences of eating food that is processed with chemicals containing inorganic mercury.

CONCLUSION

In this chapter, you learned about how vegetable oils, corn sweeteners, food colors, and preservatives are manufactured and in which foods these ingredients are most commonly found. You also learned that there are certain amounts of heavy metals, such as arsenic, lead, and mercury, that are allowed in these food ingredients. There is a significant risk of heavy metal exposure when you consume foods containing these ingredients. These metals are able to displace zinc from the metal carrier protein metallothionein (MT), and this can lead to zinc losses from the body.[2] Zinc losses adversely impact health by creating inflammation and stress.[2] Heavy metal exposures and/or low zinc status are associated with Alzheimer's disease, autism, hyperactivity, pica, type 2 diabetes, insulin resistance, and heart disease conditions.[59,60,61,62,63,64] The focus of the next chapter will be on the role of the standard American diet in creating some of these Western disease conditions.

Our Western Diet and Disease

In the previous chapter, we took a look at the processed food ingredients in vegetable oils, corn sweeteners, food colors, and preservatives. We examined how the consumption of these food ingredients can contribute to heavy metal exposures and increased risk of disease. What you eat can either help or harm your body in its mission to stay balanced and healthy, because it determines how your genes react to heavy metal and other toxic substance exposures. The quality and type of food you eat is your body's only defense against toxic substance exposures and the development of disease. So if you are enjoying good health, it is, in part, because of what you are eating. In this chapter, we will take a closer look at what Americans eat on an annual basis. We will determine if there has been a change in the types and amounts of foods eaten over the past forty years to account for the increasing prevalence of learning disorders and chronic diseases.

STANDARD AMERICAN DIET

While the chemical makeup of human genes—also known as the genome—has remained stable for centuries, what we eat has changed drastically over the last forty years.[1,2] The dietary changes have impacted the way human genes behave, making us more susceptible to disease.[2,3] In the United States, the Western diet is also known as the Standard American Diet, or SAD, and is characterized by the intake of *processed foods* containing high amounts of refined sugar, fats, oils, and refined grains.[1,3] The dietary changes that have occurred in the United States are now occurring in other countries worldwide. This widely-adopted trend began in the late twentieth century, especially after agriculture was first included in international trade rules in 1994.[4] As a result, the growth of transnational food companies has exploded and new foods have been introduced across the globe.[4]

Along with the new dietary changes, there is an increase in the number of people suffering from the so-called "Western diseases." Public health agencies are tracking the increasing prevalence of Western diseases in each country that has adopted the Western diet. In addition to neurodevelopmental disorders,[5] the Western diet is responsible for the increased prevalence of diabetes, heart disease, cancer, asthma, allergies, dementia, chronic joint disease, skin and digestive disorders, and Alzheimer's disease.[2,3] In the sections below, we review a couple of case studies of countries that are adopting the SAD and the health effects of these dietary changes.

Mexico

In 1994, the North American Free Trade Agreement (NAFTA) between the United States (U.S.), Mexico, and Canada propelled the integration of American and Mexican markets. The transition to free trade in sugar and high fructose corn syrup (HFCS) did not begin until 2007, however.[6] Soon after NAFTA, a sugar dispute erupted between Mexico and the U.S. which resulted in the restriction of sugar imports from Mexico and HFCS exports to Mexico.[6] Once the dispute was settled in 2007, Mexico's HFCS market increased from 9 percent during 2005–07 to 25 percent during 2012–14.[6]

As NAFTA was fully implemented, the U.S. began to invest billions of dollars in Mexican food manufacturing—especially for processed foods. American beverage and snack food manufacturers introduced their products and influence to the country.[4] This new relationship between the two countries saw a drastic change in the types of foods available and consumed in Mexico:

- Between 1995 and 2003, sales of processed foods (such as snacks, baked goods, and junk foods) increased by 5–10 percent every year.[4]

- From 1992 to 2002, the amount of soft drinks consumed per year spiked from 275 eight-ounce servings to 487 servings (exceeding the United States' 436 servings per year).[4]

- Meanwhile, from 1984 to 1998, purchases of fresh foods such as fruits and vegetables, milk, and meats became much less frequent, dropping by as much as 29 percent.[7]

Convenience stores and large supermarkets that provide easy access to soft drinks and snack foods started to replace small, family-owned stores.[4] The spike in availability and consumption of foods high in energy and low in nutrients contributed to the declining well-being of the people in Mexico. The overweight and obese population nearly doubled from 33 percent in 1988[4] to over 70 percent in 2012.[8] Mexico now has the highest percentage of obese citizens in a populous nation, with the U.S. a close second.[9] The 2013 *State of Food and Agriculture Report,* published by the Food and Agriculture Organization of the United Nations (FAO), blamed industrialized agricultural production, sedentary lifestyles, and the popularity and convenience of processed snacks for the rise in overweight and obese populations in industrialized and middle-income countries.[9]

It is important to note that annual HFCS consumption per person in Mexico still remains much lower than in the U.S.[6] According to a recent U.S. Department of Agriculture report (published in 2014), the average Mexican consumed about 24 pounds per year of HFCS, while the average American consumed 46 pounds per year.[6] (In Chapter 4, I had reported the average American consumed 26.8 pounds per year of HFCS in 2014. My estimate was based on USDA data made available to the public.) HFCS alone is clearly not responsible for the obesity epidemic, although it may play an important role.

In 2014, the World Health Organization determined that non-communicable diseases—the most common of which are heart disease, cancer, type 2 diabetes, and respiratory disease—were the cause of over 75 percent of the total deaths in Mexico.[10] These diseases are largely associated with poor diet. (See "Unhealthy Diet Linked to Increasing Disease" on page 81.)

China

In a similar narrative to Mexico, the prevalence of overweight and obese people in China has soared. While Mexico has become a notable consumer of soft drinks, China has become one of the largest producers and consumers of vegetable oils in the world.[4] As you learned in Chapter 4, vegetable oils often can be a source of trace amounts of mercury (which can alter gene function), as well as dietary fat (which can contribute to cardiovascular disease, among others).

New tax, import, and trade regulations in the 1990s led to the development of a relationship between China and Brazil, the world's second-largest producer and exporter of soybeans.[4] Soybean oils, and then other vegetable oils, became much more popular in Chinese cooking and diet—in 2012, China imported 9.6 million tons of vegetable oil and over 62 million tons of oilseeds (the majority of which were soybeans).[11] In the same year, 51 million tons of refined vegetable oils were produced in China (mostly in the forms of soybean oil, rapeseed oil, and peanut oil).[11] Foods manufactured with vegetable oils are inexpensive and easily accessible, especially to the poor.

The growing popularity of vegetable oils is concerning. Even Chinese government officials noticed: In 2004, a senior health official said that more effort was needed to educate the public in the face of a growing health crisis, and noted that the recommended daily intake of vegetable oil was 25 grams.[12] That year, the average daily vegetable oil consumption in China was 35.1 grams (adding an extra 180 calories per day)[13]—although it reached as much as 83 grams per day in some urban and rural areas.[12]

Over 33 percent of adults in China are overweight or obese as of 2016,[14] compared with the 11.7 percent of overweight or obese people in 1991.[15] Rising health problems range from diabetes to vitamin deficiencies to malnutrition[14] (which is a lack of important nutrients—not necessarily a lack of food).

These examples from Mexico and China reflect a growing, worldwide trend: The adoption of the Standard American Diet in the form of soft drinks, corn sweeteners, processed snacks, and vegetable oils, and the subsequent rise of obesity and other harmful health conditions. Later in this chapter, you will learn in what ways these foods interact to cause chronic health problems such as heart disease and diabetes.

UNHEALTHY DIET LINKED TO INCREASING DISEASE

The SAD is what leads to the development of the chronic disease conditions and obesity in American adults and their children. After several generations of eating the SAD, children in the U.S. are now being diagnosed with the chronic Western diseases once seen only in adults. Increasing numbers of prescriptions are being filled by physicians to treat children as young as six years of age who have conditions of hypertension, high cholesterol, and type 2 diabetes.[16]

In addition to contributing to overall inorganic mercury exposure and increasing risk of type 2 diabetes, overconsumption of corn sweeteners and vegetable oils may also lead to obesity in humans of all ages, including infants. There has long been debate about whether being overweight or obese is an inherited condition or a dietary consequence. Actually, it is a little bit of both. The obesity problem begins in our children before they are even born. We now know that as the expectant mother consumes HFCS, she is affecting and determining the lifelong function and metabolic systems of her baby.[17]

Although HFCS is considered an *obesogen*—a foreign compound that disrupts normal function and development of metabolic systems, leading to increased risk of obesity[17]—obesity is a condition of *transgenerational* malnutrition. Nutritional deficits that occur when eating the SAD impact gene regulation and function from one generation to the next.[18] What this means is that obese and overweight women will essentially give birth to babies who are metabolically programmed to become obese and more likely to suffer from chronic Western disease conditions as they age.[19]

HOW THE STANDARD AMERICAN DIET CHANGES YOUR PHYSIOLOGY

Let's go into more detail on the SAD and how it changes the way your body functions. In the previous chapter, you learned that Americans increased their vegetable oil consumption by 250 percent from 1970 to 2010 and increased their HFCS consumption by 8833 percent from 1970 to 2014. HFCS is a refined sugar and vegetable oil is a refined fat. Both ingredients are commonly found in the highly processed foods that characterize the SAD.

Previously, we had discussed the idea that inorganic mercury exposures from the consumption of these two major food ingredients may lead to zinc losses from the body. While there are no studies linking the consumption of vegetable oils to zinc loss, there are studies that show the consumption of fructose or HFCS may lead to changes in physiology that create mineral imbalance and/or losses in humans.[20,21] The mineral losses of greatest concern to me include zinc and calcium, because both of these micronutrients are crucial for preventing the Western diseases we've been discussing throughout this book.

Zinc Loss May Lead to Elevated Inorganic Blood Mercury Levels

In a 1992 study, American scientists Ivaturi and Kies determined consumption of fructose and HFCS by humans may lead to mineral imbalances, including zinc loss.[21] You may remember we have already discussed how consumption of yellow food colors leads to zinc loss in hyperactive children.[22] If your body does not have sufficient zinc because you are consuming too much HFCS, metallothionein (MT) gene function may become impaired, disrupting your ability to excrete heavy metals. The purpose of the zinc-dependent MT gene is to produce the protein metallothionein, required by your body to excrete inorganic mercury and lead from your body. Your body cannot build MT protein molecules if it does not have enough zinc atoms. Zinc loss from consuming fructose and HFCS could therefore lead to the bioaccumulation of certain heavy metals.

There is strong evidence to suggest the bioaccumulation of inorganic mercury is already occurring in the American population and creating health problems, even without considering potential zinc loss. A researcher by the name of Dan Laks analyzed blood results data collected by the Centers for Disease Control (CDC) from 6,174 American women of childbearing age.[23] The data was collected by

CDC during the 1999–2006 time period; the women ranged from eighteen to forty-nine years old. Laks found that within this population, detectable inorganic blood mercury levels rose sharply from 2 percent of the women in 1999–2000 to 30 percent of the women in 2005–2006.[23] Laks also found that the *average* detectable inorganic blood mercury levels rose significantly over the same period of time.[23] What this means is inorganic mercury accumulates over time in the body with increasing age[23] as women continue to eat the toxic Western diet. The older a woman gets, the more inorganic mercury there will be in her body if she does not change her diet.

No one has done the same kind of study to determine if average inorganic mercury levels also rise in men as they age. Studies have been conducted, however, on both rats and humans to determine how higher blood mercury levels impact health by increasing the risk of heart disease and type 2 diabetes.[24,25,26,27,28,29] Many of these same studies indicate that it isn't just mercury causing these health problems; exposure to, and the bioaccumulation of, lead and arsenic also contributes to the development of these Western disease conditions.

In Chapter 4, you learned about all of the food ingredients for which there are allowable and/or expected levels of inorganic mercury, arsenic, and lead. Highly processed foods containing food colors, sodium chemicals, preservatives, bleached flour, vegetable oils, and corn sweeteners are all potential sources of heavy metal exposure, especially inorganic mercury. We now know that mercury exposure increases the risk of metabolic disease. With respect to the development of type 2 diabetes, inorganic mercury exposure from the consumption of processed food is directly related to fasting glucose, or blood sugar levels.[30] The next section will explain how we know this.

Inorganic Blood Mercury Levels and Diabetes

In Chapter 4, I discussed a small study my collaborators and I conducted at a community college. During the study, we asked some students to eliminate corn sweeteners from their diets while we educated other students about the contaminants found in processed foods and the requirements for proper nutrition. The students who gave up corn sweeteners were given guidance on choosing and cooking food without corn sweeteners. We found that when students significantly reduced their consumption of processed foods while increasing their intake of whole, unrefined foods, they had lower inorganic blood mercury and lower fasting glucose (blood sugar) levels than students who only eliminated corn sweeteners from their diets.[30] Our findings indicated blood inorganic mercury and fasting glucose levels could be influenced by dietary intake of processed foods.[30] As students eliminated more processed foods from their diets, their inorganic blood mercury and fasting glucose levels decreased.

To confirm the relationship between inorganic mercury in blood and fasting glucose levels, we partnered with researcher Dan Laks to analyze the CDC's National Health and Nutrition Examination Survey (NHANES) dataset.[31] The NHANES dataset is used by researchers all over the world to study the roles of diet and lifestyle in the development of disease.[31] CDC collects the data from thousands of Americans who answer survey questions about their diet and lifestyle and donate blood and urine samples for analysis.[31] The blood and urine samples are analyzed by CDC to determine a wide range of *biomarker* levels.[31] Biomarkers are measureable compounds or elements found in human body tissues and fluids. The levels of certain biomarkers can help determine if a disease is present in the body, or if there is a risk of disease. See Table 5.1 below for examples. As you will see, the fasting blood glucose level that we discuss in this section can be used to diagnose the presence or risk of developing diabetes:

Table 5.1. The Biomarkers Doctors Measure to Diagnose Disease or Determine Risk of Disease

Biomarker	Disease State
Blood lead level	Developmental delay, behavioral abnormalities, lead poisoning, ADHD, autism
Fasting blood glucose level	Diabetes
Hemoglobin, hematocrit levels (blood)	Anemia
Protein in urine	Kidney disease

In our collaboration with Dan Laks, we analyzed the blood mercury and glucose measurements taken from 16,232 Americans—men and women, across all races—from 1999 to 2012.[30] The results of our analysis showed that inorganic mercury (I-Hg) detection is directly associated with fasting glucose in the NHANES 1999–2012 dataset.[30]

Our results indicated that as inorganic mercury accumulates in the blood of Americans, their fasting glucose levels also rise.[30] The results of our study also indicate that the more processed foods you eat, the higher your inorganic blood mercury and fasting glucose levels will be.[30] It goes without saying that as your fasting glucose (blood sugar level) rises, so does the risk of being diagnosed with type 2 diabetes. To avoid type 2 diabetes, it is important to reduce your intake of processed food ingredients known or allowed to contain trace amounts of inorganic mercury. The tables provided in Chapter 4 will help you determine which processed food ingredients may contain mercury. Avoid their consumption, along with corn sweeteners.

Our small study at the community college showed that it isn't enough to just eliminate corn sweeteners from the diet. To improve fasting sugar levels, one must also reduce intake of the other processed food ingredients that may contain inorganic mercury while increasing intake of whole, unrefined foods. This means that you and your family members need to eat more whole foods and less refined foods to reduce your inorganic mercury levels, fasting glucose levels, and subsequent risk of type 2 diabetes.

By now it should be clear to you that inorganic mercury exposure and bioaccumulation may occur as a result of the consumption of highly processed foods. In a dietary environment of heavy metal exposure and zinc deficiency, metallothionein (MT) protein production may be reduced, allowing mercury and other heavy metals to accumulate in blood and body tissues.[32]

DIETARY DEFICITS ADD TO DISEASE RISK

Dietary vitamin and mineral deficiencies that result from eating the Western diet are common and problematic in the U.S.[1] For example, magnesium deficiency is a characteristic of the Western diseases hypertension, heart disease, type 2 diabetes, and attention deficit hyperactivity disorder (ADHD).[33,34] In 2009, USDA scientists reported finding that almost half of all Americans over the age of one do not meet their average daily dietary requirement for magnesium.[35] More currently, the National Institutes of Health reported that dietary surveys of Americans consistently show that magnesium intake is lower than the recommended amount across all age groups.[33] In the U.S., where the average citizen consumes 46 pounds of HFCS each year,[6] these reports are especially alarming. Years ago, USDA scientists warned that when one's dietary magnesium intake is low, consumption of HFCS leads to lower calcium levels as well.[20] Lower calcium levels adversely affect the body's ability to maintain its internal balance.[20]

Calcium Deficit Problem in Children

When body calcium levels are low, calcium-dependent genes such as PON1 and BDNF may not be able to perform their jobs. As you may recall, your body needs its PON1 gene to activate and express the paraoxonase enzyme to break down neurotoxic organophosphate pesticide residues. These pesticide residues are routinely found in foods in the SAD. You also need your BDNF gene to express itself so your memories will stay intact from one day to the next. USDA scientists have warned that the consumption of HFCS may lead to calcium loss,[20] which in turn may affect the performance of PON1 and BDNF genes. This warning comes at a time when there is increasing evidence the SAD already does not provide sufficient dietary calcium. This is most worryingly a concern in children and adolescents.

Insufficiencies in dietary calcium among children in the U.S. have already been documented by scientists at the CDC.[36] CDC scientists reported in 2008 that 80 percent of adolescent girls did not eat enough foods high in calcium.[36] In addition to this finding, the scientists reported that adolescent girls reduced their milk consumption by 36 percent, while nearly doubling their average daily soft drink consumption from 6 ounces a day to 11 ounces a day.[36] These are unfortunate findings, especially since these girls may eventually become pregnant; calcium deficiency in pregnancy results in the birth of babies born prematurely or with low birth weight.[37,38] High power studies (studies in which the sample sizes are large enough to render reliable findings) have shown that babies with a low birth weight are at significantly higher risk of developing autism and ADHD.[39,40,41]

While it is important to track the dietary calcium intake of adolescent girls due to their childbearing capacity, it is equally important to determine the calcium intake of children under the age of twelve. As I mentioned in Chapter 2, adequate calcium intake is crucial to detoxify the body of lead, which is commonly found in the environment. Exposure to lead may cause brain damage and impair learning. CDC estimates that 4 million households in the U.S. have children living in them that are being exposed to high levels of lead.[42] You may be wondering by now if dietary calcium intakes in U.S. children are adequate to detoxify the lead found in their environment.

In the late 1990s, one group of scientists conducted a study of the dietary calcium intake in 314 U.S. children ranging in age from one to eight years.[43] They found that 31.4 percent of the children in the one- to three-year-old age group and 59 percent of the children in the four- to eight-year-old age group had calcium intakes below the recommended dietary guidelines.[43] This was an important study because it raised a red flag indicating that dietary calcium intake among young children in the U.S. may be too low for proper gene regulation and function and for metabolizing and excreting lead from the body.[43,44] Remember from Chapter 2 that children with ADHD and pervasive developmental delay (PDD) tend to accumulate lead in their bodies, and this may be due to a diet deficient in calcium.[43,44,45,46]

Because we are seeing an increasing number of children in the U.S. being diagnosed with ADHD, autism, and PDD, it is important to consider the changes in the American diet that might explain the reductions in calcium intakes among children. I have extracted data from the USDA food availability system and determined these changes for you. Table 5.2 on page 88 shows the changes in the consumption of foods rich in calcium over the last forty years in the U.S. The foods included in the analysis are those that are free of added sugars and relatively high in calcium compared with other foods. The data is adjusted for loss or spoilage so it more nearly reflects actual consumption.[47]

Table 5.2. Consumption of Calcium-Rich Foods in the United States

Commodity	1970 per capita Consumption (lbs/year)	2012 per capita Consumption (lbs/year)
Almonds	0.3	1.5
Broccoli, fresh	0.21	2.50
Broccoli, frozen	0.6	1.59
Cheese, cheddar	4.8	7.9
Cheese, Swiss	0.42	0.52
Fish, salmon, canned	0.5	0.1
Fish, sardine, canned in oil, drained	0.2	0.1
Milk, total, plain, whole and lower fat, unflavored	178.6	107
Peas, frozen	1.26	1.19
Raisins, seedless	0.88	0.85
Yogurt, refrigerated	0.6	9.8
Spinach, fresh	0.14	0.73
Spinach, frozen	0.31	0.39
TOTAL	**188.82**	**134.17**
Percent decrease in consumption of calcium-rich foods 29%		

From my analysis of the data provided in the table above, it appears that over the last forty years Americans have reduced their overall consumption of healthy calcium-rich foods by 29 percent. I believe this reduction in dietary calcium and the increased intake of HFCS are important factors in the development of neurodevelopmental disorders such as ADHD and those found in the autism spectrum. I believe calcium deficiency is also related to hypomethylation, which is associated with certain other Western diseases (see "Declines in Methyl-Donating Food Intake" on page 89). Although there are no human studies available to support my belief, scientists recently reported that pregnant rats fed a diet deficient in calcium gave birth to hypomethylated pups.[48]

Declines in Methyl-Donating Food Intake

Remember from Chapter 2 that hypomethylation—the shortage of methyl groups in the body—is a characteristic of the following disease conditions: Autism, type 2 diabetes, Alzheimer's, heart disease, atherosclerosis, and hypertension. When diets are deficient in methyl-donating foods, hypomethylation may occur in addition to calcium deficiency. A variety of foods are known to be rich in methyl groups. Any reduction over time in the intake of these foods could certainly explain some of the hypomethylation we are seeing in conjunction with the Western diseases. In writing this book, I thought it would be important to determine if there have been any changes in the American dietary intake of methyl-donating foods.

Because the USDA food availability system does not collect consumption data for *all* foods high in methyl group-donating nutrients, determining these changes for you proved to be difficult but not impossible. I was restricted to collecting only the data that was available from the USDA food availability system. The data I have prepared in Table 5.3 was adjusted for loss or spoilage and reflects actual consumption of the listed foods containing methyl group-donating nutrients.[47]

From my analysis of the data provided in Table 5.3 on page 90, it appears that over the last forty years, Americans have reduced their overall consumption of foods high in methyl-donating nutrients by approximately 20 percent. I believe this reduction in intake of methyl-donating nutrients—combined with the decrease in calcium intake—is a factor in the increasing prevalence of diseases associated with hypomethylation.

In Chapter 2, we discussed the role of methyl groups in gene regulation and function. It is crucial for the family diet to include foods that contribute methyl group-donating nutrients. Study after study shows that children with autism and ADHD and adults suffering from type 2 diabetes, hypertension, fatty liver, obesity, and heart dis-

Table 5.3. Consumption of Methyl Group-Donating Foods in the United States

Commodity	1970 per capita Consumption (lbs/year)	2012 per capita Consumption (lbs/year)
Beef	60.9	41.7
Broccoli, fresh	0.21	2.50
Broccoli, frozen	0.60	1.59
Chicken	22.4	46.2
Eggs	23.9	19.0
Fish, canned, salmon	0.5	0.1
Milk, plain, whole and lower fat, unflavored	178.6	107
Peppers	0.79	4.26
Shellfish, fresh/frozen	1.3	2.7
Spinach, fresh	0.14	0.73
Spinach, frozen	0.31	0.39
Total tree nuts	1.4	3.2
Turkey	4.0	7.9
Veal	1.2	0.2
TOTAL	**296.25**	**237.47**

Percent decrease in consumption of methyl group-donating foods 20%

ease all suffer from nutritional deficiencies that can be traced back to the inadequate intake of foods that provide essential methyl group-donating nutrients.[49,50,51,52,53,54] Methyl groups are needed by the body to turn the genes on that produce the proteins and enzymes required to rid the body of environmental toxins that are associated with the development of these disease conditions. Mercury, pesticides, lead, and arsenic are all examples of the toxicants found in your family's environment every day. Exposure to these toxicants may occur in the air you breathe, the water you drink, and especially the foods in the SAD you may eat. It is so important to avoid and manage these exposures by adopting a healthy diet that will improve your health status; your health status is a reflection of what you eat.

A HEALTHY DIET TO IMPROVE YOUR HEALTH STATUS

A healthy diet consists primarily of whole, organic, pesticide-free foods. Such a diet does not include highly processed foods containing the ingredients and toxicants discussed in this book (vegetable oils, corn sweeteners, food colors, preservatives, and pesticide residues). To improve your health status, you will want your diet to mostly consist of the following foods:

- Organic vegetables and fruits
- Cold-pressed olive oil
- Nuts
- Organic whole grains
- Legumes
- Low-fat dairy
- Low-mercury fish
- Grass-fed beef
- Chicken

In this chapter, I've provided lists of foods high in calcium and high in methyl group-donating nutrients. You will need to incorporate these foods into your daily diet. In Chapter 8, I will provide additional lists of healthy foods, including fish, and discuss the value of supplements.

CONCLUSION

In this chapter, we've discussed how the unhealthy Standard American Diet (SAD) increases the prevalence of Western diseases, including type 2 diabetes, heart disease, hypertension, Alzheimer's, ADHD, and autism. Many of the foods in the SAD introduce toxicants, such as inorganic mercury and lead, to your body, and these exposures change the body's physiology. Mineral imbalances occur as a result and provide mechanisms for disease or disorder development. The American diet has changed over the past forty years and these changes have resulted in critical deficits in important minerals such as zinc, calcium, and magnesium. These mineral deficits, along with reductions in the consumption of methyl-donating foods, have made the typical American more susceptible to developing disease. In the next chapter, we will discuss the consequences of the SAD on our society's children.

6.

———

Spotlight on Autism and ADHD

In the previous chapters, we identified the foods we need to include in the family diet and the food ingredients we need to eliminate to ensure proper gene function. We learned that methyl-donating nutrients play an important role in turning genes on and off. We determined the importance of essential micronutrients that are lacking in the Western diet, and learned that many food ingredients are sources of heavy metal and/or pesticide exposures. By now, we hopefully have a better understanding of the role the Western diet plays in creating conditions for the development of common Western diseases, including autism, ADHD, type 2 diabetes, neurodegenerative disorders, and heart disease.

In this chapter, we will briefly discuss the increasing prevalence of autism and ADHD in the United States. Then I will explain how the toxic substances in the food supply may impact gene function and contribute to risk factors that lead to the development of these debilitating conditions. We will explore the roles and costs of prevention or treatment. We will discuss how healthy dietary interventions can work to reduce symptoms, and the side effects of the most common ADHD medications will be explored.

INCREASING PREVALENCE OF AUTISM AND ADHD

The Centers for Disease Control and Prevention (CDC) has been tracking the occurrence, or *prevalence,* of autism and other developmental disabilities in the U.S. population since 2000.[1] Autism is defined by the American Psychiatric Association (APA) as a disorder that affects brain development and impacts social and communication skills.[2] It appears within a child's first three years of life.[2] The occurrence of autism varies according to location, gender, and environmental conditions. For example, in New Jersey, 1 out of every 41 eight-year-olds has autism, while in South Carolina the prevalence is 1 out of every 81 eight-year-olds.[1]

Consider the following statistics on the prevalence of autism in the U.S.:

- Boys are 4.6 times more likely than girls to be diagnosed with autism.[1]

- CDC estimates the prevalence of autism in the U.S. population has increased 123 percent from 2002–2010.[1]

- The number of children ages six through twenty-one receiving special education services for autism increased 91 percent between 2005 and 2010.[3] My collaborators and I reached this conclusion by reviewing special education data maintained by the U.S. Department of Education.[3]

Although estimated prevalence varies depending on the study design and data collected, it is clear the number of children with autism is increasing in the U.S.

The number of children with attention deficit hyperactivity disorder, or ADHD, is rising in the U.S. as well. The APA defines ADHD as a behavioral condition in which staying focused and getting organized are challenging.[4]

Consider the following statistics on the prevalence of ADHD in the U.S.:

- In a 2014 article, CDC scientists estimated the prevalence of ADHD in the U.S. to be 11 percent of all children aged four to seventeen years.[5]

- The CDC scientists also reported in 2011 that, compared with 2003, 2 million more U.S. children had been diagnosed with ADHD.[5]

- The CDC reported that the rate of ADHD diagnosis increased by 5 percent each year between 2003 and 2011.[6]

● As is the case with autism, boys are more likely than girls to be diagnosed with ADHD.[6]

ADHD prevalence also varies by location. For example, in Nevada, 5.6 percent of all children have been diagnosed with ADHD; in Kentucky, 18.7 percent of all children have been diagnosed with ADHD.[6] Diet is considered among scientists to be an *environmental factor* in the development of ADHD. In previous chapters, we discussed the role of diet in creating conditions for ADHD. Remember that deficits in dietary calcium lead to the bioaccumulation of lead—which is a factor in the development of ADHD—and food color consumption can lead to zinc loss, which accompanies hyperactivity (a defining trait of ADHD). In the next section, we will delve more into the causes of autism and ADHD.

ROOT CAUSES OF AUTISM AND ADHD

Most scientists now agree the root causes of autism and ADHD are related to gene-environment interactions associated with toxic substance exposures, either in the mother's womb or after the child is born. A child's genes respond to environmental factors, including diet and toxic substance exposure, and this creates conditions for the development of autism or ADHD. There are several competing theories about the etiology (cause) of autism and ADHD, but each has some connection to the environment. A search on PubMed, the U.S. government database which maintains all officially recognized medical journal articles, revealed between 10,000 and 13,000 articles which discuss the causes of autism and ADHD.[7,8]

Some scientists provide evidence that mercury exposure is the cause of autism. For example, families living downwind from a coal-fired power plant that releases mercury emissions are at increased risk of having a child with autism.[9] In one study, scientist Richard Palmer found that for each 1,000 pounds of mercury released to the environment, there was a 61 percent increase in the rate of autism and a 43 percent increase in the rate of special education in Texas.[9] Other researchers point to lead, pesticides, or some other toxic substance exposure as the contributor to or cause of autism and ADHD.

Spotlight on Vaccine Controversy in Autism

The vaccine theory of autism began in 1998 with a single publication in the British medical journal *Lancet*.[10] The publication, written by Andrew Wakefield and twelve others, suggested that the development of pervasive developmental delay (PDD; a form of autism) was linked to the measles, mumps, and rubella (MMR) vaccination.[10] In 2000, a group of parents in the U.S. founded the non-profit advocacy organization named SafeMinds[11] to promote the vaccine theory,[12] fund research to find evidence supporting the vaccine theory,[13] and educate others about the harmful side effects of vaccines containing ethylmercury or thimerosal.[14]

According to the FDA, however, thimerosal was never used as an ingredient in the MMR vaccine in the U.S.[15] Furthermore, it has been many years since thimerosal was reduced to trace levels in or removed from vaccines recommended for children.[15] The Centers for Disease Control (CDC) continues to track the increasing number of children with autism in the U.S. and indicates on its webpage that thimerosal is not a factor in the development of autism.[16,17]

The CDC funded nine different studies; each showed no relationship between vaccination or thimerosal and the autism epidemic.[17] With the exception of the flu vaccine, thimerosal was removed from vaccines between 1999 and 2001,[17] yet autism rates continue to climb each year in the U.S.[16] From 2000 to 2012, the CDC determined the prevalence of autism in eight-year-old children increased from 1 in 150 to 1 in 68.[16]

Meanwhile, the publication by Wakefield et. al in 1998 was completely retracted by the *Lancet* in February 2010.[10] Apparently, Wakefield falsified data for the purpose of financial gain.[10] The author's research had been funded by lawyers representing parents in lawsuits against vaccine companies.[10] It is unlikely Wakefield's coauthors knew of the fraud. Ten of the coauthors published their own retraction in the *Lancet* in 2004, writing, "no causal link was established between MMR vaccine and autism as the data were insufficient."[18] Wakefield has since lost his license to practice medicine.[19] Despite the fraudulent publication and evidence to the contrary, many parents still continue to believe vaccines are the cause of autism.

SafeMinds is not the only parent group concerned about the safety of child vaccines. In 2005, Generation Rescue was founded by the parents of a child who developed autism after receiving several vaccinations along with antibiotics.[20] Its mission is to support the recovery of children with autism by providing parents with guidance and support for medical treatment.[20] This is the organization currently led by Jenny McCarthy, an actress and talk show host.[20] Generation Rescue works to provide parents with resources and facts on nutrition, vaccination, and information about the latest scientific findings on the cause and prevention of autism.[21] The organization also provides grants to parents who are struggling financially to pay for the biomedical treatments needed by their children to recover from autism.[22] Generation Rescue works collaboratively with the National Vaccine Information Center (NVIC), the oldest vaccine safety group in the U.S.

NVIC was founded by parents of vaccine-injured children in 1982 and its mission is to prevent vaccine injuries and deaths.[23] NVIC is the biggest consumer-led organization in the U.S. advocating for patient informed consent and vaccine safety.[23] NVIC does not advocate for or against the use of vaccines. The organization simply believes parents have a right to know the risks of harm associated with vaccination and the right to choose whether or not to vaccinate their children.[24]

Vaccine injuries do occur and it is my belief that it is a parent's right to choose when or whether they vaccinate their children. I allowed healthcare providers to vaccinate my children in the early '80s before thimerosal was removed from vaccines. In those days, there were fewer recommended vaccinations than there are today. How often a child receives recommended vaccines is referred to as the *childhood immunization schedule.* Today's immunization schedule is far busier than the one I followed for my children in the early '80s.

In my opinion, it would be wise for parents today to follow a slower-paced immunization schedule than is currently recommended so there is enough time for their child to recover between individual vaccinations. Parents can judge for themselves when their child is ready for the next vaccine. I do not think vaccines are the cause of autism. I do believe, however, that a vaccination may contribute to the development of autism in genetically predisposed individuals under certain circumstances, such as the consumption of a poor prenatal diet, exposure to toxic substances, and/or poor infant feeding practices.

Despite the various theories, the truth is that there is no *single* cause of autism or ADHD. At this point, we cannot know the cause of either condition in any given child. What we do know is that in many children, dietary pattern can improve or worsen the symptoms of each disability. This chapter is a discussion of the environmental factors associated with autism and/or ADHD that you can control to some degree through family diet.

Many people believe vaccines are the cause of autism. Please see the "Spotlight on Vaccine Controversy in Autism" inset starting on page 96 to learn more about this controversial issue.

PESTICIDE EXPOSURE IS A RISK FACTOR

In previous chapters, we discussed at length the evidence that shows toxic metal exposures from processed food consumption contribute to the development of both learning disabilities and Western disease. In Chapter 3, we discussed the role of pesticide exposure in adult-onset neurological diseases such as Alzheimer's disease and Parkinson's disease. By now, you are probably wondering if there is any evidence to suggest that pesticide exposures also contribute to the development of autism, ADHD, and pervasive developmental delay (PDD).

Indeed, there are numerous published studies that show that organophosphate (OP) pesticide exposure, both before and after the birth of a child, is associated with the development of autism, ADHD, and PDD.[25,26,27,28,29,30,31,32] Intuitively, you must know the pesticide residues most frequently found in the foods we eat are likely the very ones responsible for the rising prevalence of neurodevelopmental disorders. We will now review a couple of the studies that show your intuition is correct.

Pesticides and ADHD

A Canadian scientist by the name of Maryse Bouchard led a fairly recent study to determine which OP pesticide is more closely related to the development of ADHD.[25] She and her team analyzed the CDC data collected from the National Health and Nutrition Examination Survey (NHANES). The data was collected during the four years for which ADHD was assessed in American children eight to fifteen years of age.[25] Bouchard et al. assumed the 1,482 children under study in the general population were getting their OP pesticide exposure primarily from fruits and vegetables.[25] It really doesn't matter where the children got their pesticide exposure from, however. When the researchers analyzed the urinary metabolite output data for the children, they found the metabolite levels for malathion exposure were much higher in the children diagnosed with ADHD compared with the levels in the children in the general population who were not diagnosed with ADHD.[25]

Bouchard's study shed light on the impacts of OP pesticide exposure on a child's ability to learn *after* the child is born. Exposure to malathion when a child eats conventionally grown wheat, corn, fruit, and vegetables is clearly a factor in ADHD. Symptoms of ADHD include fidgeting, tapping one's hand or feet, running around inappropriately, leaving a seat in the classroom when sitting is the expected behavior, inability to pay attention or follow directions, and demonstrating a lack of patience when waiting for one's turn. All of these symptoms may impact a child's ability to learn in the classroom setting.

These symptoms may be reduced when a child's malathion exposure is eliminated or significantly decreased through the adoption of an organic, pesticide-free diet. In fact, researchers have found that children with ADHD show significant improvement in many areas by switching to an organic diet.[33,34] CDC scientists have confirmed that if you feed your child organic foods, you will significantly lower his dietary exposure to OP pesticides.[35] If your child has been diagnosed with ADHD, you can help him learn better by switching to an organic diet. More information about organic foods can be found in Chapters 7 and 8.

Pesticides, Autism, and Developmental Delay

Prenatal pesticide exposures occurring *in the womb* appear to be more closely linked to the development of autism and developmental delay (DD)[26] in children after they are born. In a recent study, conducted by researchers in California led by Janie Shelton, prenatal exposures to pesticides were determined by the mothers' residential proximity to agricultural operations and fields prior to and throughout the pregnancy period.[26] Geographical pesticide application data was obtained from the California Pesticide Use Report.[26] Shelton and her team compared the state pesticide application data to the residential proximity data provided by parents of 486 children with autism, 168 children with DD, and 316 typical or "normal" children.[26]

Basically, where a mother lives—her address—is a factor in determining her overall exposure to pesticides and risk of giving birth to a child with autism or DD. Exposure to the OP pesticide chlorpyrifos during the second trimester and nonspecified OP pesticides during the third trimester was closely linked to the development of autism.[26] Meanwhile, exposures to carbamate pesticides (see inset on page 101) were more closely associated with DD.[26] The take-home message here is that proximity to OP pesticides at some point during pregnancy increases risk of autism in the child by at least 60 percent.[26]

The closer a pregnant woman lives to an agricultural operation that applies pesticides on its crops, the more likely it is she will be exposed to harmful pesticides. It is important to note that Shelton et al. did not consider *dietary* pesticide exposures in their study.[26] Exposures were presumably via inhalation (air contaminants) and possibly via ingestion (dust). Once again, however, it really doesn't matter where the pesticide exposure came from. The important point is that when pesticide exposure occurs, it is significantly associated with the development of the neurodevelopmental disorders that are increasing in prevalence. What you can do if you are an expectant mother is adopt an organic diet and reduce your child's overall exposure to pesticides in the womb. The science-based evidence tells us that we must eliminate or significantly reduce the expectant mothers' pesticide exposures to have the best possible birth and child development outcomes.

In the case of OP and carbamate pesticide exposures, whether the exposure is via food or inhalation or before or after birth, a child's body must have the ability to metabolize and eliminate the pesticides via urinary output. Good health outcomes are related to having this

Carbamate Pesticides

In previous chapters, we discussed organophosphate (OP) pesticides and the damage they can do to the genes that are responsible for eliminating toxic substances from your body. Another type of pesticide we mention in this chapter is the carbamate pesticide. Although their chemical makeup is different, carbamate pesticides work in a similar manner as the OP pesticides; they are used for killing insects in the home and in agricultural fields.[37] Inhaling or ingesting carbamate pesticides can inhibit an enzyme in your nervous system called acetylcholinesterase, damaging your nerve function.[37,38] As mentioned on page 100, prenatal carbamate pesticide exposure has been linked to developmental delay in children.[26]

ability.[35] The most important player in the game of pesticide residue elimination (especially in the case of organophosphate pesticides) is the PON1 gene.[36]

PON1 GENE EXPRESSION SUPPRESSORS

As we mentioned in Chapter 2, the PON1 gene is calcium-dependent and responsible for carrying the instructions for producing paraoxonase (PON), an enzyme which the body must have in order to break down and eliminate organophosphate pesticide residues. This is why it is so important for the family diet to contain enough calcium! Any substance known to reduce calcium intake or interfere with calcium metabolism should be avoided.

The PON1 enzyme is made in the liver with calcium and secreted in the blood, where it is incorporated into high density lipoproteins (HDL). Overconsumption of any substance that impacts liver function, such as alcohol or high fructose, will suppress PON1 gene activity and lead to disease conditions.[36] While the exact mechanism of PON1 gene suppression is not known, years ago, USDA scientists warned that when dietary magnesium intake is low, consumption of high fructose corn syrup (HFCS) leads to lower calcium levels.[39] When body calcium levels are low, the calcium-dependent PON1 may not be able to perform its job. Since the availability and activity of PON1 are impaired in many children with autism and ADHD,[40,41] it is thus important to limit their exposures to any substance known to further suppress PON1, making them even more susceptible to the toxic effects of OP pesticide residues.

The bottom line is that children with autism and ADHD need to avoid consuming foods that may lead to calcium losses, including fructose and HFCS. In the case of pregnant women, we know that if their PON1 gene activity is low, they will be more likely to give birth to a child with ADHD.[42] For this reason, pregnant women also need to avoid consuming foods known to lead to calcium losses. It goes without saying that by avoiding dietary pesticide exposures in the first place, many of these disease conditions can be avoided.

With respect to PON1 gene activity, it is important to note that in addition to alcohol and high fructose, we know of other factors that modulate, or alter, the gene's expression.[36,43] The most important factors, in my opinion, are inorganic mercury and lead exposures.[36,43] From previous chapters, we now understand that inorganic mercury and lead exposures occur daily through the consumption of highly processed foods. These particular heavy metal exposures may suppress PON1 gene activity.[36,43] In the case of inorganic mercury, we know that as we get older and continue to eat the toxic Western diet, our inorganic blood mercury levels will rise[44] and our PON1 gene activity will fall. I believe the loss of PON1 gene function is one reason why older people are more prone to developing Western diseases such as Alzheimer's, type 2 diabetes, cancer, and heart disease.

PON1 GENE EXPRESSION IN CHILDREN

What about our children? PON1 gene activity plays an important role in the body's developing immune system. Age is the most important factor of all, as PON1 activity is very low before birth and gradually increases during the first few years of life in humans.[43] In one study, scientists at UC Berkeley found the PON1 activity levels in many children may remain lower than those of their mothers for several years.[45] The scientists concluded that these children may be more susceptible to OP pesticides throughout their childhood and more vulnerable to developing autism.[45] Gender matters, too. Baby boys are born with lower PON1 activity compared to baby girls.[36,43] The lower PON1 activity in boys certainly explains why they are at far greater risk of developing autism and ADHD than girls! They have less capacity to produce the paraoxonase enzyme and are more susceptible to the adverse effects associated with OP pesticide exposure.

In a different study, scientists at UC Berkeley found that two-year-old children were less likely to display symptoms of developmental delay when their mothers had higher PON1 gene expression during their pregnancy.[46] Proper function and adequate expression of the PON1 gene is essential both for prenatal development and child health because exposure to OP pesticides is a common occurrence in the U.S. It is therefore important for the family diet to be free of contaminants that may suppress PON1 gene activity, such as inorganic mercury,[36,43] lead,[47,48] and high fructose corn syrup![36]

WHAT DOES OP PESTICIDE EXPOSURE LOOK LIKE?

If a child with low PON1 gene activity eats food, such as wheat end products, laced with OP pesticide residues, he is going to have a reaction. The symptoms he feels will be similar to those experienced by someone with a low or underactive thyroid.

Both low and high levels of exposure to OP pesticides impact thyroid function in adults who have low PON1 gene activity.[49] We can certainly expect the same or greater impact on thyroid function in children with low PON1 gene activity when they are exposed to OP pesticide residues and cannot break down the pesticide residues in their food supply. The result is OP pesticide poisoning, which is often misdiagnosed by pediatricians as respiratory infection, viral syndrome, gastroenteritis, atopic dermatitis, or drug-related encephalopathy.[50] Children with low PON1 gene activity, especially those diagnosed with autism or ADHD, may exhibit any of a number of symptoms (listed on page 104) associated with low thyroid and/or OP pesticide poisoning.[50,51]

Symptoms of Thyroid Dysfunction or OP Pesticide Poisoning

- Cognitive dysfunction (anxiety, memory deficits, depression)
- Cold intolerance
- Constipation
- Drowsiness, lethargy, fatigue
- Dry skin, dermatitis
- Gastroenteritis, intestinal abnormalities

- Growth retardation
- Headache
- Increased infections
- Seizures or rigidity
- Slow speech or speech impairment
- Weight gain or difficulty in gaining weight

MATERNAL OBESITY AND DIABETES AS RISK FACTORS

In Chapter 4, we learned the average American was consuming 35.6 pounds of corn sweetener, including 26.8 pounds of HFCS, per year in 2014. Several studies now link excess sugar consumption with the development of obesity, and fructose is thought to somehow play a special role.[52] No one disputes the fact that excess sugar consumption leads to obesity. There is, however, a disagreement between the Corn Refiners Association (which represents the HFCS industry), the sugar producers, and many in the scientific community over the *type* of sugar most responsible for obesity.

In my view, excessive intake of all types of sugars is a risk factor for obesity and should be avoided by any woman wishing to become pregnant. There is abundant literature available now to support the hypothesis that maternal obesity significantly increases the risk of autism, ADHD, and other neurodevelopmental disorders in children.[53] In a 2016 human study, scientists found that obese pregnant women in the U.S. were significantly more likely to have a child with ADHD after ten years of follow up.[54] In other studies, scientists found that obese pregnant women with gestational diabetes (a form of diabetes that develops during pregnancy) are more likely to produce a child with autism.[55,56]

HFCS consumption may well play a role in the obesity and autism epidemics. My collaborators and I published a paper in the *Behavioral and Brain Functions* journal in 2009 showing that the net growth in persons diagnosed with autism in California matched the net growth of per capita HFCS consumption from 1987–2006.[57] Notably, from 2000–2002, the rate of autism diagnoses peaked at 19.6 percent, while annual per capita HFCS consumption peaked at 44.8 lbs/year. After 2002, both the rate of autism diagnoses and the annual per capita HFCS consumption fell.[57]

Although we were lucky to find datasets during that time period for the variables of "autism cases" and "per capita HFCS consumption,"[57] we did not even consider the important factor of maternal obesity. We were more focused on HFCS consumption, which we now know is only part of the story. It is not unusual for scientists to restrict their research to a confined area of concern or to have competing theories as to why a disease occurs. But such tunnel vision, along with the lack of interdisciplinary research, is the reason why we have not solved the chronic disease problems we continue to see today.

Nonetheless, HFCS consumption is even more concerning now because recent evidence suggests that its consumption by an expectant mother may contribute to her baby's risk of becoming an obese adult. A rat study published in 2016 confirms that maternal intake of high fructose leads to metabolic programming in the fetus that results in adult obesity, hypertension, and metabolic dysfunction, leading to heart disease.[58] What this suggests for humans is that as each generation becomes more obese, we will continue to see increasing prevalence in autism, hypertension, type 2 diabetes, and heart disease. When babies are born with the programming to become obese, we must do all we can to prevent this situation from occurring.

In addition to avoiding sugar and HFCS during pregnancy, one thing a woman can do to prevent her baby from becoming obese is avoid feeding him baby formula. We will discuss the reasons why in the next section.

BABY FORMULA AND OBESITY, AUTISM, AND ADHD

Scientists have reported in recent medical journal articles that babies that consume formula are at higher risk of becoming obese.[59,60] In the U.S., infant obesity is considered to be an epidemic by the government.[61] Recent estimates indicate that 8.1 percent of American infants and toddlers are obese.[61] What is even more disturbing and controversial is the finding that formula feeding may significantly increase a child's risk of autism.[62,63] You may wonder what food ingredients found in infant formula might contribute to obesity or autism. Figure 6.1 below is a reproduction of a food ingredient label for an infant formula that I found available for purchase in a supermarket.

INGREDIENTS: 42.6% corn syrup solids, 14.7% soy protein isolate, 11.5% high oleic safflower oil, 10.1% sugar (sucrose), 8.4% soy oil, 7.8% coconut oil, 2.4% calcium phosphate; less than 2.0% of: C. cohnii oil, M. alpina oil, potassium citrate, sodium chloride, magnesium chloride, ascorbic acid, L-methionine, potassium chloride, choline chloride, taurine, ferrous sulfate, ascorbyl palmitate, m-inositol, zinc sulfate, mixed tocopherols, L-carnitine, niacinamide, d-alpha-tocopheryl acetate, calcium pantothenate, cupric sulfate, thiamine chloride hydrochloride, vitamin A palmitate, riboflavin, pyridoxine hydrochloride, beta-carotene, folic acid, potassium iodide, potassium hydroxide, phylloquinone, biotin, sodium selenate, vitamin D3 and cyanocobalamin.

CONTAINS SOY INGREDIENTS.

Figure 6.1. Baby formula food ingredient list.

Many baby formulas, such as this one, contain corn sweetener in the form of corn syrup or corn syrup solids. Some formulas contain more corn sweetener than any other ingredient! I found one baby formula product in my local grocery store with a food ingredient label that claimed 54 percent of the product was made up of corn syrup solids and 26 percent of the product consisted of assorted vegetable oils. With many baby formulas consisting of this mixture of sugars and fats, it is no wonder that babies fed on formula are at a higher risk of becoming obese.

The baby formula pictured on page 106 and many other formulas contain multiple vegetable oils. Remember from Chapter 4 that vegetable oils are among the food ingredients that are at risk of inorganic mercury contamination. Exposure to this heavy metal can affect the PON1 and metallothionein gene expressions.

Below is a table of common ingredients found in infant formula and the heavy metal(s) with which each ingredient can potentially be contaminated.

Table 6.1. Common Ingredients Found in Infant Formula and Potential Heavy Metal Contaminants

Ingredient	Heavy Metal Contaminant
Coconut oil	Mercury (Hg)
Corn syrup or corn syrup solids	Mercury (Hg)
Palm oil	Mercury (Hg)
Soybean oil	Mercury (Hg)
Sunflower oil	Mercury (Hg)
Vegetable oil	Mercury (Hg)
Potassium chloride	Lead (Pb)
Beta carotene	Lead (Pb), Arsenic (As)

This table of baby formula ingredients is not all-inclusive. I studied the food ingredient labels of only six different formula products. There could be other risky ingredients; there are many more producers out there making baby formula.

You may now be wondering: Have scientists determined the levels of heavy metals in infant or baby formula? The answer is yes. Numerous studies have been conducted by scientists all over the world to determine the level of heavy metal contaminants in baby formula. Some very recent studies have identified higher than allowable levels of mercury in baby formula.[64,65,66] In one study, two of three formula samples contained mercury in concentrations over 120 times above the allowable weekly limits.[64] The researchers, based in the Philippines, warned of the possible direct or cumulative effects of these mercury exposures on infant health.[64]

In another study, two of three infant formulas were again found to contain mercury in concentrations above the allowable weekly intake.[65] These researchers were based in Libya and they published their results in 2015.[65] In a third study, published in 2012, researchers in the European Union obtained formula samples from twenty-four different formula makers and found that while lead levels were within the "safety limits," mercury levels were not.[66] These scientists, based in Germany, warned the mercury accumulation occurring in some formula-fed infants would be higher than the established weekly tolerable intake.[66] Canadian researchers also investigated mercury levels in baby formula and found clear cases of mercury contamination in powdered formula.[67] The Canadian researchers discovered one brand of concentrated liquid infant formula had significantly higher mercury levels than other liquid brands.[67]

The only study published in the U.S. on heavy metal contamination of baby food or infant formula was conducted by FDA researchers, and they only looked at arsenic contamination in products made from rice, as well as fruits and vegetables.[68] In Portugal, researchers determined statistically significant differences for mercury content between processed organic and conventional baby cereal products.[69] Apparently, organic baby food contained less mercury than conventional baby food.[69] No surprise finding there, as organic food is produced with no synthetic pesticides.

To minimize her baby's heavy metal exposure and risk of obesity, a mother could opt to eat a healthy, organic, whole-foods diet and breastfeed. A study found that babies fed only formula or fed a combination of breast milk and formula are more likely to become obese compared with babies who are only breastfed.[59] The age at which breastfeeding stops and formula is introduced also appears to be a key determinant of obesity risk throughout childhood, adolescence, and even young adulthood.[60] Numerous scientists are therefore recommending to new mothers that they exclusively breastfeed for at least six months to protect their infants from becoming obese or autistic.[60,62,63,70,71] Sometimes, there are situations in which mothers are unable to breastfeed. I advise any mother who is feeding formula to her baby to buy and use an organic brand to minimize the baby's heavy metal exposure.

AUTISM AND ADHD PREVENTION OR TREATMENT

In this chapter, we've discussed at length the most likely root causes of autism and ADHD; they all lead back to improper diet and the poor quality of the food supply. In previous chapters, we've discussed at length how poor diet and inadequate nutrition impair or disrupt gene function and the body's ability to remove toxic substances. Child behaviors associated with autism and/or ADHD have been linked to food color consumption; elevated lead, mercury, or other heavy metals in blood; hypomethylation (see inset below); insufficient dietary calcium; zinc losses; gene variation, suppression, or dysfunction; and other toxic substance exposures, including pesticides, alcohol, and cigarette smoking. Each of these factors may contribute to the development of behaviors associated with autism and ADHD. So what can you do to prevent or even treat the symptoms of autism or ADHD?

Hypomethylation

Recall from Chapter 2 that hypomethylation occurs in children who have autism. Hypomethylation is when the body does not have enough methyl groups to turn on certain important genes, such as brain derived neurotrophic factor (BDNF, which promotes learning and memory). Eating methyl group-donating foods (such as foods high in methionine, choline, and folic acid) can help combat hypomethylation.

Adopt a Healthy Diet

Some parents have found that adopting a healthy family diet can bring about positive changes in the afflicted child's behavior; this can reduce or eliminate the need for costly intensive behavioral supports. While dietary improvements have been shown to reduce poor behaviors in some children with autism or ADHD,[33,34,72,73,74,75,76,77] healthy diet alone will not cure these conditions in the more severe cases. The older a child is, the greater the accumulation of toxic substances in his body, and this toxic load will increase the severity of his symptoms. The younger a child is diagnosed, the better his chances of healing through healthy diet.

When eliminating toxic substances from the child's diet *does* work, there is no going back to the old, poor dietary pattern. These children often have difficulty eliminating toxic substances due to genetic variation or gene dysfunction, and this metabolic condition is permanent. It will not simply go away, so they must abstain from eating highly processed or pesticide-laden foods that expose them to toxic substances. The more the toxic substances build up in their systems, the more challenging their behavior becomes. The children must be kept free of toxic substances to maintain their bodies' balance.

Medication

In the case of children for which adopting a healthy diet does not work, medication is the treatment of last resort in my view. The decision of whether or not to medicate a child who has behavioral difficulties is a hard one for most parents. Unfortunately, many physicians are not trained in nutrition or diet,[78,79] so children and their families are never given the opportunity or encouragement to try dietary changes first. Only 25 percent of medical schools require their medical students to take a dedicated nutrition course.[78] In the conventional medicine setting, prescription medication is therefore almost always the first line of defense in treating both autism and ADHD. Off-label prescription medicines (medicines prescribed for uses other than what the FDA has approved) are used commonly to treat autism, and Ritalin is used frequently to treat symptoms of hyperactivity in children with autism and ADHD. Unfortunately, Ritalin is a controlled substance (meaning its use is regulated by the government) because it can be abused or lead to dependence.[80] According to the FDA, Ritalin has many side effects, including sudden death in patients with heart problems.[80] Reported side effects of Ritalin are presented on page 111.

Side Effects of Ritalin[80]

- Circulation problems (e.g. numbness in fingers or toes, skin color changes, sensitivity to temperature)

- Decreased appetite

- Dependence or addiction

- Eyesight changes

- Headache

- Increased blood pressure and heart rate

- Interactions with other medications (e.g., cold or allergy, blood pressure, blood thinner, seizure, or anti-depressants)

- Nausea

- Nervousness

- New or worse aggressive behavior or hostility

- New or worse behavior and thought problems

- New or worse bipolar illness

- New psychotic symptoms or new manic symptoms

- Seizures

- Slowing of growth (height and weight) in children

- Stomachache

- Stroke and heart attack in adults

- Sudden death in patients with heart defects or heart problems

- Trouble sleeping

Prevention Versus Treatment

The CDC, scientists, some governments, and other public health entities recommend eliminating toxic substance exposures from the child's environment, including from the diet, before and after they are born. It is easier and less costly to prevent the conditions of autism and ADHD than to treat them:

- In 2011, CDC estimated the public health costs for children with autism in the U.S. to be up to $60.9 billion per year.[81]

- More recently, the annual cost for autism in the U.S. in 2015 was estimated to be $268 billion.[82]

- According to the CDC, intensive behavioral interventions for *one* child with autism costs between $40,000 and $60,000 per year.[81]

● The public health cost for children with ADHD in the U.S. was estimated in 2007 to be significantly less, at $42.5 billion per year on average.[83]

If the prevalence of autism continues to grow as it has, treatment costs for autism will far exceed those associated with diabetes (estimated in 2014 to cost $322 billion per year[84]) by 2025.[82] As a former public health service officer, it would seem to me that the public health goal in the U.S. at this point in time should be to provide dedicated nutrition and health education to young people at an early age so that by the time they reach childbearing age, they have adopted clean and healthy diets. Such a strategy will lead to reductions in the number of cases of autism and ADHD. Another important strategy for tackling the problem would be to eliminate toxic substances from the food supply.

CONCLUSION

By now, I hope you have a whole new view of autism, ADHD, and the factors that contribute to these debilitating conditions, which jeopardize the quality of life and learning for a significant portion of our nation's population. In Chapter 8, I will provide specific guidance for creating a safe food environment in your home.

In the meantime, there are many things you can do as a parent or relative of a child afflicted with autism or ADHD. You can encourage the proper feeding of the child so that he has a healthy diet rich in the calcium required to support proper PON1 gene function. The child's diet also must contain adequate zinc, to build the metallothionein proteins that metabolize and excrete heavy metals (such as inorganic mercury and lead) that make it into the food supply (refer back to Chapter 2 for more details). You can encourage the elimination of food ingredients from the family diet that suppress PON1 gene activity, such as high fructose corn syrup or those ingredients that are allowed to contain heavy metals. Such ingredients include those we discussed in Chapter 4 and the ingredients included in some baby formulas, listed in Table 6.1. The child's family can switch to organic produce and food products to reduce their overall exposures to pesticides. If a baby is being fed formula, the family should seek an organic brand. If the baby is breastfed, the mother should take care to eat nutrient-rich foods that are free of pesticides or heavy metals.

In the case of autism, the evidence suggests that day-to-day hypomethylation may be corrected in part by increasing the intake of foods high in methyl group-donating nutrients, while at the same time reducing exposures to environmental toxins found in the food supply, such as inorganic mercury and organophosphate pesticides.[85,86] In the next chapter, I will provide information on reading food ingredient labels to help you avoid toxic substances in the food supply. You will also learn about how the FDA and food industry's version of "safe" substances came to be.

7.

Food Labeling Practices

In the previous chapters, we identified how you may become exposed to toxic heavy metals or pesticides by eating foods commonly found in the Standard American Diet (SAD). Such exposures may directly interfere with gene function or promote the development of disease through essential mineral losses (e.g., zinc, calcium) that impact body metabolism. We discussed some of the common diseases associated with these exposures, including type 2 diabetes, autism, ADHD, heart disease, and neurological diseases such as Alzheimer's.

In this chapter, we will cover some topics that often come up when consumers are trying to make the best food choices while grocery shopping. We will briefly discuss the FDA and the food manufacturers' roles in food ingredient safety and labeling practices, how food ingredients are determined to be "generally recognized as safe," food ingredient labeling requirements, food marketing practices, natural versus organic foods, the gluten-free diet, and concerns about dietary supplements.

It is important to acknowledge at the onset that food labels are deceptive in their marketing, and this is how toxic substances enter our food supply. The labels omit trace contaminants and processing chemicals that the Food and Drug Administration (FDA) does not require to be listed. Meanwhile, controversial and harmful food ingredients, such as high fructose corn syrup, are listed because the FDA has granted such ingredients a "generally recognized as safe" status.

Before beginning our look into food labels, we must first look at the founding and relevant history of the agency that regulates food labeling practices—the FDA.

ESTABLISHING THE FDA

The FDA came into being with the passage of the 1906 Pure Food and Drug Act by Congress.[1] The 1906 Act was passed in response to the public's outrage at the filthy conditions of the Chicago stockyards (livestock storage areas) and meatpacking factories, described by Upton Sinclair in his book *The Jungle*.[1] With the establishment of a consumer protection agency, Congress hoped to reduce the misconduct that was happening in food manufacturing.[1]

In addition to establishing the FDA, the 1906 Act sought to ban the addition of food ingredients that would conceal damage or be harmful to consumers' health.[2] The Act stated that labels on food and drugs could not be misleading in any way. According to the FDA, the Act's main objective was "the regulation of product labeling, rather than pre-market approval."[2] In other words, the law focused on the *accuracy* of food labels; the food ingredients themselves did not have uniform standards, as long as they were not outright harmful.[2] The famous "snake oil" scam is one early example of the role the Act played in enforcement. (See inset below.)

Snake Oil's Exposure by the 1906 Act

The term "snake oil" is used today to mean a product (especially a medical substance) that is promoted as a remedy, but has little or no real value. This definition originated when a man named Clark Stanley began selling his rattlesnake oil product, claiming it to be legitimate, effective Chinese snake oil rich in omega-3 acids,[3] and marketing it as a cure-all. After the 1906 Pure Food and Drug Act was passed, a shipment of Stanley's Snake Oil was analyzed and found to contain no snake oil at all—instead, it was a combination of mineral oil, red pepper, and turpentine. It had no healing effects. As per the 1906 Act, Stanley was fined for misbranding and misrepresenting his product—not because of the safety of the ingredients themselves.[3]

FDA AND USP'S ROLES IN INGREDIENT SAFETY

Prior to 1906, there was no U.S. government food or drug safety regulatory agency. Instead, there was the private U.S. Pharmacopeial Convention (USP), which began setting standards for drug and ingredient quality in 1820.[4] In those days, "ingredients" included the therapeutics of the time—tonics, extracts, honeys, infusions, liniments, mixtures, ointments, pills, syrups, vinegars, extracts, powders, wines, and so on.[4]

Today, the USP is a scientific, non-profit, trade organization made up of volunteers and individuals working in various regulated industries. The organization sets standards for the identity, strength, quality, and purity of medicines, food ingredients, and dietary supplements. These products are manufactured, distributed, and consumed worldwide.[5] USP only recently took over the food ingredient safety standards from the National Academy of Medicine (formerly the Institute of Medicine).[5]

As a consumer, it is important to understand that FDA has always adopted the food ingredient and drug safety standards set forth by trade organizations such as the USP or other likeminded organizations. The U.S. Congress gives FDA the authority to codify and enforce these standards to protect public health. According to its website, FDA's responsibilities include regulating food, cosmetics, dietary supplements, drugs, and vaccines to ensure that these items are safe, effective, and properly labeled.[6] Many consumers do not realize that FDA is only an enforcement agency; it does not determine whether or not a food ingredient is safe. Organizations like the USP set those standards. The responsibility of making sure a food ingredient meets those standards lies in the hands of food manufacturers. The FDA determines if the food manufacturers are following the rules.

THE GRAS PROCESS

Manufacturers are required to determine if a food ingredient is safe. Does this mean that the safety of food ingredients on the market today has already been determined through evidence or science-based research? Actually, it does not.

For many years, FDA never required food manufacturers to demonstrate that their food ingredients were safe.[7] Prior to the 1950s, there were few food ingredient safety standards or laws in the U.S.[7] In 1949, FDA commissioner Paul B. Dunbar initiated a Congressional investigation of some of the chemicals used in food.[7] For two years, the investigation went on and recommendations were made to change the existing food and drug laws to impact the use of certain food additives and colors.[7] Most of the changes to the food laws were outlined in the Food Additives Amendment enacted by Congress in 1958.[8] For the first time, no substance could legally be introduced into the U.S. food supply unless there had been a prior determination of its safety by the manufacturer.[7] This is the landmark act in which Congress had essentially assigned the task of determining the safety of food ingredients to the food manufacturers.[7]

In passing the 1958 Food Additives Amendment, Congress gave FDA the authority to determine which of the hundreds of food ingredients already on the market could be considered "Generally Recognized as Safe," or "GRAS," and exempt from further review by FDA.[8] What FDA did next amounted to grandfathering.

FDA published the first "list" of food ingredients meeting the GRAS criteria in 1958.[8] The ingredients that achieved GRAS status and made it onto the GRAS list could be used *without restriction* in food products. They were considered safe—not because they had undergone any formal evaluation or study to determine their toxicity on human health, but because they already had a long history of use in food.[8] The substances on the first GRAS list were essentially grandfathered in to the new system of determining food ingredient safety. Additional food ingredients were placed on the GRAS list only after the manufacturer submitted a petition to the FDA. In many cases, food ingredients had been on the market for many years without a safety determination, but had not made it onto the first GRAS list. Despite this, the ingredients continued to be allowed in food products. We will now look at high fructose corn syrup (HFCS) as a case study to see how a food ingredient may be placed on the GRAS list through the petition process, which continues to this day.

How HFCS Was Determined "Safe"

In 1983, after high fructose corn syrup (HFCS) had already been on the market for several years, the corn refining industry submitted a petition to FDA to consider HFCS a safe substance because it was made from enzyme preparations that FDA had already recognized as GRAS. Additionally, HFCS was thought to be the same as honey, with minor components found at levels similar to those in corn syrup and corn sugar—substances that were also already on the GRAS list.[9]

FDA approved the petition submitted by the corn refining industry, not because HFCS had been studied to determine any adverse impact on human health, but because the substance was similar in makeup to other substances already considered safe.[9] With respect to the potential harm to sensitive subpopulations, FDA reviewers wrote that the requirement to list "high fructose corn syrup" on the ingredient label was warning enough to sensitive consumers.[9]

In 1996, despite objections from a diabetes research center, FDA reaffirmed its decision to consider HFCS a GRAS substance.[9] Of course, today there is ample evidence to show the harm of HFCS consumption to human health, both in terms of contributing to obesity and the development of type 2 diabetes. Yet, HFCS remains on the GRAS substance list and can be used as a food ingredient without restriction or warning to consumers of its potential adverse health effects.

GRAS Database

FDA provides a database of some of the hundreds of GRAS substances.[10] Of the food ingredients we've talked about in this book that are detrimental to your health, several are considered to be generally recognized as safe by the FDA. This means they can be added to food without restriction. The most common ingredients found on food product labels are listed in Table 7.1 on page 120, along with their allowable impurity levels or their known risk of heavy metal contamination.

What is missing from this table? In Chapter 4, we discussed the mercury cell caustic soda (sodium hydroxide) and hydrogen chloride used routinely to regulate the acidity, or pH, of food products

Table 7.1. GRAS Ingredients with Allowable Heavy Metal Impurities or Likely to Contain Heavy Metal Contaminants

Ingredients	Allowable Heavy Metal Impurities	Likely to Contain Metal
Calcium chloride	Lead ≤ 2 ppm	
Caramel	Arsenic ≤ 3 ppm Lead ≤ 10 ppm Mercury ≤ 0.1 ppm	
Citric acid	Lead ≤ 0.5 ppm	
Potassium chloride	Lead ≤ 2 ppm	
Sodium benzoate	Lead ≤ 2 ppm Mercury ≤ 1 ppm	
Sodium diacetate	Lead ≤ 2 ppm	
Corn syrup		Mercury (Hg)
Dextrose (corn sugar)		Mercury (Hg)
High fructose corn syrup		Mercury (Hg)
Potassium chloride		Lead (Pb)

≤ means less than or equal to

during the manufacturing process. Remember, these substances contain trace amounts of inorganic mercury that may bleed into the food supply, creating an exposure hazard to consumers who eat highly processed foods. These substances will not be listed as a "food ingredient" on labels like the ingredients in the first column of Table 7.1 would be listed. In my view, if these substances are allowed to contain trace amounts of mercury, then they, too, should be listed on the food ingredient label as processing aids. A mercury warning label should also be applied to the packaging. The consumer has a right to know *all of the chemicals* that were used to produce each food product.

In this climate of limited regulation, consumers must have access to all of the information regarding processed foods. Remember in Chapter 5, we established the fact that the more processed food your family eats, the higher their blood inorganic mercury levels may be. We learned that higher blood mercury levels increase your risk of heart disease, diabetes, and other Western diseases. What would be optimal for reducing chronic Western diseases at this juncture would be to ban substances with allowable trace mercury or other heavy metal levels entirely from the food supply. At a minimum, they should definitely no longer have GRAS status. Without GRAS status, restrictions would be placed on when and how much of the substances can be used. It is so important for you, as a consumer, to read and understand food ingredient labels so you can minimize your exposures to the toxic substances in our food supply!

FOOD LABELING REQUIREMENTS

Food labeling is regulated in the U.S. by the FDA. Food manufacturers are required to follow the package labeling guidelines provided by the FDA.[11] FDA does not pre-approve each food label, but provides guidance to manufacturers on *what* they need to include on packaging.[11] With respect to the ingredients in a food product, FDA requires the manufacturer to list each ingredient in descending order of predominance by weight.[12] What this means is the ingredient that weighs the most is listed first, and the ingredient that weighs the least is listed last.[12] Whether or not exposure to an ingredient becomes toxic over time is beside the point. For example, trace or incidental amounts of mercury, lead, arsenic, or pesticides are not required to be listed on the food ingredient label. The FDA has no definition of how much a "trace amount" is, and the FDA also does not require ingredients that have "no functional or technical effect in the finished product" to be listed.[13] Certain food allergens are the exception to the rule on "trace amounts."

Food Allergen Labeling

The only time a trace amount of an ingredient must be listed on the food package label is when it is considered a "major food allergen."[12] Of the more than 160 food allergens known to cause reactions in sensitive individuals, FDA recognizes eight of them.[12] If any of the following eight "major food allergens" may be present in the food product, then FDA requires manufacturers to either list them in the ingredient list or in a "contains" statement[12]:

1. Crustacean shellfish

2. Egg

3. Fish

4. Milk, including whey

5. Peanuts

6. Soybeans

7. Tree nuts

8. Wheat

The table below illustrates the two different ways trace amounts of the "major food allergens" can be listed on the food label:

INGREDIENTS: Whole wheat flour, water, high fructose corn syrup, corn syrup, egg, soybean oil, whey, yeast, sugar, soy flour. **Contains:** Milk, soy, egg, wheat.	INGREDIENTS: Whole wheat flour, water, high fructose corn syrup, corn syrup, egg, soybean oil, whey (milk), yeast, sugar, soy flour.
Label 1	Label 2

The labels in the table are also examples of highly processed foods. A highly processed food is one that has been changed from its whole, natural state. The more processed a food is, the more food ingredients you will see manufacturers list on the label.

Other Labeling Requirements

In addition to a list of the food ingredients, manufacturers must provide other information on the food package label, such as nutrition facts and manufacturer contact information.[11] Manufacturers may also indicate whether their product meets the criteria for the "organic" designation, and they may make FDA-approved health claims.[11] Organic foods must be produced without the use of pesticides and cannot contain pesticide residues. This is different from foods labeled "natural" or "made from natural ingredients." FDA has no official definition for "natural" and so cannot enforce the use of this term. Even a highly processed food or a food that has been produced with pesticides could be labeled "natural."[14]

To the average consumer, the food package label appears straightforward. However, the reality of the situation in our industrialized society is far different than you might imagine. While food labels do provide some good information about the product found inside the package, they are also used as marketing tools for manufacturers.

FOOD MARKETING PRACTICES

The marketing of food is the same today as it was 200 years ago. We live in a "snake-oil society," where manufacturers often make health claims that may not help consumers distinguish healthy food choices from less healthy food choices. Many claims made by manufacturers on food packaging are, indeed, false or misleading.[15] One recent FDA commissioner wrote an open letter to manufacturers stating the following problem: "Misleading 'healthy' claims continue to appear on foods that do not meet the long- and well-established definition for use of that term."[15]

In addition to claiming food is healthy when it is not, manufacturers also use labels for marketing purposes to mislead and prompt consumers to buy products they may not even need. "Gluten-free" labels placed on products today are an excellent example of misleading marketing practices used by food manufacturers.

"Gluten-Free" Marketing

Gluten is a protein found in wheat, barley, and rye.[16] Individuals with the inherited chronic inflammatory autoimmune disorder known as *celiac disease* have difficulty metabolizing gluten. Their bodies think gluten is a dangerous, foreign substance, and their immune systems declare war. Symptoms of an irritable bowel may ensue upon exposure to wheat. The stricken individuals may feel cramping, abdominal pain, bloating, gas, or experience diarrhea or constipation. A properly trained gastroenterologist can easily diagnose whether or not a person truly has celiac disease.

Anybody who has been diagnosed with celiac disease would do well to eat a diet of gluten-free foods. However, the term "gluten-free" has also become a marketing tactic to entice people who do not have celiac disease into spending more money on a product they have been led to believe is healthier.

FDA currently allows food manufacturers to voluntarily label any product "gluten-free," as long as the product contains less than 20 parts per million (ppm) gluten.[17] This means any—and I mean *any*—product meeting the less than 20 ppm gluten criteria can be labeled "gluten-free." Foods that are by nature gluten-free, such as bottled water, may be labeled "gluten-free."[17] This is not considered "misleading" marketing by the FDA because, technically, these items are indeed gluten-free. But by placing a "gluten-free" label on a product, the consumer is led to believe the food normally must have gluten; otherwise, why would one manufacturer apply the "gluten-free" label on the package, while another does not?

A study published in 2016 in *JAMA* examined results from the National Health and Examination Surveys (NHANES) from 2009–2014.[18] The study found that between the years of 2009 and 2014, the percentage of people who followed a gluten-free diet—but did not have celiac disease—more than tripled.[18] Meanwhile, over the same time period, the percentage of people who had been diagnosed with celiac disease stayed about the same.[18]

The study's lead researcher, Dr. Hyun-seok Kim, said the reasons why people without celiac disease would follow a gluten-free diet include "wider availability…of gluten-free products, the diet becoming 'trendy' for health-conscious people, and [self-diagnosis] by those hoping to alleviate gastrointestinal symptoms."[19]

Many food manufacturers have noticed this uptick in the number of people who will purchase a gluten-free product without having celiac disease. A study published in the *Canadian Journal of Dietetic Practice and Research* compared unit costs of food products labeled "gluten-free" with prices of comparable gluten-containing food products. The researchers determined that on average, gluten-free products were 242 percent more expensive than regular products.[20]

The selling of a gluten-free product for which consumers will pay a higher price is attractive to food manufacturers who want to make as much money as possible. A consumer sees "gluten-free" on the label of a product and buys the product at a higher price than the same product being sold by a different manufacturer without the "gluten-free" words on the label. The product may not even be at risk of containing gluten! At the grocery store, I once saw a "gluten-free" label on coconut syrup selling at a much higher price than a competitor's product with the very same ingredient. Coconut is not a grain and is naturally gluten-free. The manufacturer was trying to add value to its product by placing the words "gluten-free" on the label. It only makes sense for the manufacturer to voluntarily place the "gluten-free" words on a product label when the food (such as wheat) truly contains gluten, but has been processed to remove the gluten.

Unfortunately, due to marketing practices or misguided advice, many parents of autistic children have put their children on a gluten free or gluten free-casein free (GFCF) diet, only to be disappointed when their children did not respond positively to the dietary changes. (Casein is a protein found in milk.) Child behavior or health outcomes will not change in response to dietary changes if the hypothesis is wrong. Gluten sensitivity or allergy is clearly not the problem in autism, unless the child is actually allergic to wheat or has celiac disease.

Spotlight on Gluten and Autism

Gluten-free food manufacturers are raking in the bucks[21,22]—sales of gluten-free foods reached $11.6 billion in 2015[23]—as they target their marketing practices at parents of children with autism,[24] despite the fact that there is no evidence to suggest a gluten-free diet will cure or alleviate symptoms of autism. On the contrary, the scientific evidence suggests the GFCF diet might actually be detrimental to child health.[25,26,27,28]

How do I know gluten-free food manufacturers are targeting parents of children with autism? I visited the "Gluten Free & Allergy Friendly Expo" website, sponsored by gluten-free food manufacturers, and read the following sentence in its mission statement: "The

Gluten Free & Allergen Friendly Expo is dedicated to meeting the needs of the celiac community, those with gluten and food sensitivities, autoimmune/inflammatory diseases, and *autism*."[24] This statement implies that gluten consumption and autism are linked. I also visited the website of one of the most well-known organizations that provides information to parents of children with autism; there, I found several gluten-free manufacturers listed as sponsors of the organization.[29]

Pushing highly processed foods—which may cause more harm than good—to parents of children with autism is disturbing to me. This is because the more processing that occurs in food manufacturing, the more likely a food will be contaminated with something unhealthy. For example, additional processing to remove gluten from grain may introduce inorganic mercury to the product if the *chemical method* is used to remove the gluten. How? The chemical method may utilize caustic soda, including mercury cell, to maintain the food product's pH during the gluten extraction process.[30] In using mercury cell caustic soda during the chemical method, trace amounts of mercury residue could end up in the final gluten-free product.

Eating gluten free products could actually lead to the bioaccumulation of inorganic mercury, which can lead to disease or make symptoms of disease worse (such as the case with autism). With or without mercury residue, the extra step in processing will make the gluten-free product more expensive and justify the higher price. Eating a gluten-free diet has risks for everybody, especially for children who have autism, as you will read in the next section.

The Problem with Gluten-Free

There are risks associated with adopting a gluten-free diet; I would not recommend undertaking such a diet unless your doctor prescribes it. Several studies now indicate that eating a gluten-free or GFCF diet may very well result in lower protein, folate, calcium, and/or vitamin D intakes, potentially risking overall health—especially in the case of autism.[25,26,27,28] Scientists recently conducted a study and found that when they fed gluten (and casein) to one group of children with autism, there was no significant difference in gastrointestinal symptoms compared with another group of children with autism, who did not eat the gluten and casein.[31] Other studies show there simply is not sufficient evidence to support the gluten-free or GFCF diet as a treatment for autism.[32,33]

Remember in Chapter 6 that we learned the symptoms that may be experienced when a child has low PON1 activity and is exposed to organophosphate (OP) pesticide residues in wheat.[34,35,36] *Many of these same symptoms are those that accompany a gluten allergy.* If a child with autism has these symptoms (see page 104), then the first line of treatment should be to take him off of any foods likely to contain OP pesticides. If his PON1 activity is low, his symptoms should disappear when he is no longer exposed to OP pesticides in conventionally grown grains, fruits, and vegetables.

When I taught special education, I worked with a child with autism. His parents thought he had a gluten allergy, but when they adopted a healthy, organic diet that was free of toxic substances, they found he could eat organic grain without any adverse effects. Once the parents stopped feeding the child gluten-free grain products along with other highly processed foods, he got better. He made significant improvements in his behavior with the healthy, organic whole food diet.

PON1 gene dysfunction as a result of poor diet is probably far more common than celiac disease, which is considered rare (impacting only about 1 percent of the population[37]). While low PON1 gene activity is common in children with autism and ADHD, a true celiac disease diagnosis is not. If your child has *not* been diagnosed with celiac disease or wheat allergy by a qualified physician, I hope you choose to buy an organic grain product instead of one claiming to be gluten-free.

It is important for you to understand that, by law, gluten-free manufacturers cannot make the health claim on food packaging that gluten-free products will cure or be of beneficial use in treating children with autism.[11] To make this claim, they would have to have FDA approval, which they do not have.[11] If you have a child with autism, please be wary of the marketing practices used by some manufacturers to persuade you to buy their products.[38,39,40] The same cautionary practice needs to be applied to the purchase of dietary supplements.

SUPPLEMENTS

The beneficial effect of using individual dietary supplements (often in the form of pills) remains unknown in most cases. Generally, they should not be taken as a replacement for healthy foods. For example, calcium supplements are advertised as potentially reducing the risk of osteoporosis. We actually know that calcium supplementation does *not* prevent osteoporosis and can increase the risk of heart attack in women by 20 to 40 percent.[41] We also know that overconsumption of various herbal and dietary supplements leads to liver injury.[42] This is not surprising, given the fact that supplements are highly processed and often contain trace amounts of heavy metals.[43] One study found that over 30 percent of dietary supplement products contain a detectable amount of mercury, while over 50 percent contain a detectable amount of lead.[43] This heavy metal contamination can come from the raw materials and plant products used in the supplements, environmental pollutants, processing factory conditions, or fillers and additives that are purposely added to the products.[43] Remember that the society we live in today allows manufacturers to sell almost anything to anyone with limited oversight and little regulation over health claims.

Dietary supplement manufacturers and distributors are not required to obtain approval from FDA.[44] FDA does not determine the safety of supplements before they are put on the market.[44] Before a manufacturer markets a supplement, the manufacturer is responsible only for ensuring the product is "safe."[44] There is no FDA oversight to ensure the manufacturer has actually conducted a safety review or study to determine any adverse effects associated with consumption of the supplement. Manufacturers are also responsible for reporting serious problems with their products to the FDA.[45] Consumers can document complaints with the FDA, as well.[46] The FDA can then pull the product from shelves if it is found to be harmful or its claims are misleading.[45] However, harmful effects can be prevented in the first place by testing and approving all products for safety *before* they are marketed and sold to consumers. There continue to be numerous supplement products on the market that confer little benefit except in specific cases. I do not recommend the use of supplements in place of whole, organic food, except in rare cases, which I will discuss in Chapter 8.

CONCLUSION

The food industry today is poorly regulated because FDA allows food manufacturers to lace our foods with toxic substances. Trace amounts of toxic heavy metal and pesticide residues left in food products kill single-celled bacteria and fungi (mold). These residues are not listed on the food ingredient label, but are hidden inside of the food ingredients themselves or the chemicals used in the food manufacturing process. As a consumer, you must be vigilant in reading food ingredient labels to determine which food products are safe to buy so you can reduce your exposure to toxic substances. Toxic substance exposures can be avoided if you stay away from foods with harmful food ingredients on the label or made with conventionally grown crops.

When processed food product packaging includes a food ingredient label, the safest product to buy is one made with organic ingredients, as well as with the least amount of ingredients. For example, the organic wheat flour pictured at right only has one ingredient. Although it must be kept in the refrigerator in a sealed plastic bag to prevent mold and insect eggs from hatching, it will not be a source of pesticide or heavy metal exposure. The fewer ingredients listed on the label, the better. The product in Figure 7.1 at right is a safe purchase. In Chapter 8, I will provide more tips and explain how you can create a safe food environment in your home.

Nutrition Facts

Serving Size 24g
Servings per Container 12

Amount Per Serving

Calories 140   Calories from Fat 40

% Daily Value

Total Fat 4.5g	7%
Saturated Fat 0.5g	3%
Trans Fat 0g	
Polyunsaturated Fat 1g	

	Calories:	2,000	2,500
Total Fat	Less than	65g	80g
Saturated Fat	Less than	20g	25g
Cholesterol	Less than	300mg	300mg
Sodium	Less than	2,400mg	2,400mg
Total Carbohydrate		300g	375g
Dietary Fiber		25g	30g

Calories per gram:
Fat 9 · Carbohydrate 4 · Protein 4

INGREDIENTS: ORGANIC WHOLE WHEAT FLOUR.
CONTAINS: WHEAT.
MAY CONTAIN: MILK.

Figure 7.1. A food product with a short ingredients list, indicating that it is minimally processed.

8.

Creating a Safe Food Environment at Home

In this book, we've talked at length about toxic substances, such as heavy metals, fructose, and organophosphate pesticides, and learned how exposures to them can occur through the contaminated foods we eat. We've learned that co-exposures to these toxic substances can lead to adverse health outcomes. To create a safe food environment in your home, you will need to eliminate foods from your diet that may contain contaminants that can become toxic over time as they accumulate in your blood and body tissues. A safe food environment is directly related to food quality. The quality of food is determined by its level of contamination and ability to provide your body with the nutrients it needs to maintain good health. Higher-quality foods contain few or no contaminants and provide your body with essential nutrients.

In creating a safe food environment, you only need to keep on hand in your kitchen the high-quality foods that enable you to consume the three major macromolecules required to maintain good health—lipids, proteins, and carbohydrates. In this chapter, we will discuss each macromolecule in detail and the best dietary sources for obtaining them. At the same time, we will discuss the role of these "food groups" in providing the nutrients and methyl-donating groups important for proper gene function. Before concluding the chapter, we will briefly discuss food allergies. All of the combined information should allow you to establish a safe and healthy food environment in your home.

HEALTHY DIET GUIDELINES

The United States government provides guidelines for a healthy diet.[1] I have revised them a bit to reflect current findings in the medical literature. A healthy diet should include the following:

- A variety of vegetables (dark green, red and orange, beans, peas, starchy)

- Whole fruits

- Whole grains

- Fat-free or low-fat dairy (e.g., milk, yogurt, cheese)

- Variety of protein foods (e.g., fish, seafood, lean meats and poultry, eggs, legumes (beans and peas), and nuts, seeds, and soy products)

- Healthy lipids

I have created a healthy diet food pyramid to serve as a visual aid so you can see how much of each type of food to eat (see Figure 8.1 on page 133). At each level of the pyramid, there are examples of appropriate foods.

At the bottom of the pyramid are examples of foods containing good carbohydrates. Your carbohydrate intake each day may be up to 65 percent of your total food intake.[2]

In the middle section of the pyramid, I have provided examples of foods rich in protein. Your daily intake of protein should not exceed 35 percent of your total diet, according to the National Academy of Medicine.[2] If you are vegetarian, it is recommended that you eat complementary proteins, such as beans and rice (also listed in the pyramid), along with tofu and nuts to supplement your protein intake.

If you eat a daily diet that provides nutrients from a variety of whole foods, you should meet your body's need for healthy lipids (fat). Lipids are placed at the top of the pyramid. Although you should eat these foods less frequently than protein or good carbs, lipids are still important for a balanced and healthy diet. Examples of foods high in good fat are provided in the pyramid (e.g., fish, avocado, walnuts, flaxseeds, olive oil).

Notice what is missing from this pyramid: Refined foods. There are only a couple of refined foods listed at the top of the pyramid, where

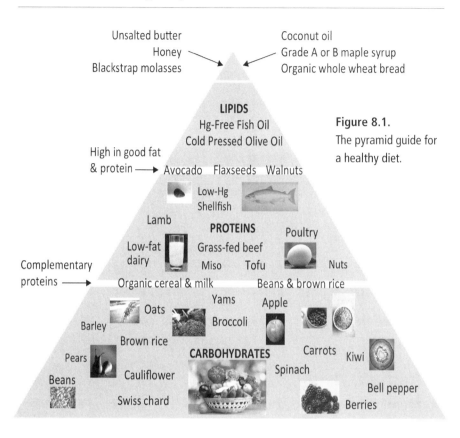

Unsalted butter
Honey
Blackstrap molasses

Coconut oil
Grade A or B maple syrup
Organic whole wheat bread

LIPIDS
Hg-Free Fish Oil
Cold Pressed Olive Oil

High in good fat
& protein ⟶ Avocado   Flaxseeds   Walnuts

Low-Hg
Shellfish

Lamb

PROTEINS
Poultry

Low-fat
dairy   Grass-fed beef

Complementary
proteins ⟶   Organic cereal & milk

Miso   Tofu   Nuts

Beans & brown rice

Oats

Yams   Apple

Barley   Broccoli

Brown rice

Pears   **CARBOHYDRATES**   Carrots   Kiwi

Cauliflower   Spinach

Beans

Bell pepper

Swiss chard   Berries

Figure 8.1.

The pyramid guide for a healthy diet.

I have provided examples of sweeteners and fats that should be consumed only in small amounts. The most refined food in the pyramid is whole wheat bread; I recommend only one slice a day, if that.

In the sections below, I will discuss the importance of each of the food groups shown in Figure 8.1 in more detail. I will also provide recommendations of dietary sources for these food groups.

LIPIDS (FATS)

Lipids are large molecules made up of fatty acids. About 90 percent of dietary fats come in the form of fatty acids.[3] Dietary fats are important sources of energy and provide the components needed to build the membrane around each cell.[3] The primary function of the cell membrane is to control the flow of matter in and out of cells.[3] Without this function, cells could not survive and reproduce. The cells in your body reproduce again and again to form the tissues of your body.

Dietary fats can be saturated or unsaturated. (See "The Molecular Structure of Lipids" below for details on the compositions of saturated and unsaturated fats.) Your intake of saturated fats should be limited. The fatty foods you eat should instead be high in unsaturated fatty acids, which can have health benefits such as reducing your risk of heart disease and lowering your cholesterol and blood pressure.[4] The unsaturated fatty acids most important for sustaining health are the omega-3 and omega-6 fatty acids.

Some tissues in your body are very rich in fat and require more omega-3 fatty acids for construction. For example, brain tissue requires more omega-3 fatty acids than heart or liver tissue in mammals.[5] The most important omega-3 fatty acid is docosahexaenoic acid (DHA), and this is why you now see DHA added to milk, eggs, and other food products. Another essential omega-3 fatty acid is eicosapentaenoic acid (EPA). Americans are deficient in their omega-3 fatty acid intake.

Dietary Recommendations for Fats

Low-fat diets may adversely affect health and lead to the inadequate intake of the important essential omega-3 fatty acids, which your body needs to survive. Experts in nutrition advise that it is far more

---

The Molecular Structure of Lipids

The fatty acid macromolecules consist of a chain of carbon atoms with a methyl group attached at one end and an acid group at the other.[3] The number of hydrogen atoms on each carbon atom determines whether the fat is saturated or not; saturated fats contain more hydrogen atoms.[3] Trans fats are unsaturated fats that have hydrogen atoms artificially added to them.[6] In unsaturated fatty acids, some of the hydrogen atoms have been replaced with double bonds between the carbon atoms.[3] The only difference between omega-3 and omega-6 fatty acids is the location of the double bond.

important to change the *type,* rather than the amount, of fats being consumed to prevent obesity and heart disease.[3] Evidence suggests that increasing your intake of omega-3 fatty acids will lower your risk of heart disease if you also decrease your intake of saturated fats and eliminate your intake of trans fats.[3] Trans fats are found in hydrogenated vegetable oils and are now considered to be detrimental to health.[7] Such oils were invented by man and have been saturated with hydrogen atoms so they will have a longer shelf life.[8]

Below is a list of foods to avoid. These foods are high in saturated or trans fats, according to the National Cancer Institute and the FDA.[9,10]

Foods high in saturated fat

- American or yellow cheese
- Burgers
- Dairy desserts
- Fried chicken
- Grain-based desserts
- Pizza
- Reduced (2 percent) fat milk
- Sausage, hot dogs or franks, bacon, ribs

Foods high in trans fat

- Baked goods (cookies, pies, cakes, crackers)
- Coffee creamer
- Fried foods (French fries, fried chicken, doughnuts)
- Margarine
- Ready-to-use frostings
- Refrigerated dough products (biscuits, cinnamon rolls, frozen pizza)
- Snack foods (potato chips, microwave popcorn)
- Vegetable shortening

In comparing the foods listed above, do you see that most are highly processed? Reducing your consumption of highly processed foods not only decreases your intake of harmful fats, but also reduces your exposures to the toxic substances we've discussed throughout this book. Consuming more whole foods and fewer processed foods will increase your intake of the important omega-3 fatty acids. Below is a list of foods high in the essential omega-3 fatty acids. Many fish and shellfish species are high in omega-3 fatty acids. Increasing your intake of these and the other foods listed below will reduce your risk of heart disease and improve brain function.

Whole Foods High in Important Omega-3 Fatty Acids

- 100 percent cod liver oil (in oil form, not pill form)
- Anchovies (fresh or canned in water)
- Catfish (caught from a clean stream)
- Clams (fresh or canned in water)
- Crab (fresh or canned in water)
- Dried algae (minimally processed)
- Eggs (with DHA)
- Flax seeds
- Grass-fed animals
- Leafy vegetables
- Oysters (fresh or canned in water)
- Salmon (fresh or canned in water)
- Shrimp
- Trout (caught from a clean stream)
- Walnuts

As you can see, I've listed cod liver oil, which is viewed as a supplement. I generally do not recommend the use of dietary supplements, but 100 percent cod liver oil is an excellent source of DHA and should be incorporated into fruit and vegetable smoothies for individuals at risk of severe omega-3 fatty acid deficiency. Such individuals often include those suffering from neurodevelopmental or neurodegenerative disorders (e.g., autism, ADHD, Alzheimer's).[11,12] Both cod liver oil and algae are equivalent sources of the omega-3 fatty acids that everyone needs to stay healthy.[13]

Notice that larger fish, such as albacore tuna or swordfish, are not listed above, even though they are high in omega-3s. I have not listed these foods because they are known to contain *organic* mercury at levels unacceptable to the developing child, fetus, and pregnant woman.[14] Please see the "Mercury in Fish and Child Development" section below to learn more about this issue and how it can affect child development.

Mercury in Fish and Child Development

There is a significant difference between the inorganic and organic mercury species (see page 19) and how each impacts human health through gene-environment interactions. We are only just beginning to understand a few of these interactions,[15,16,17] and as a result, we know very little about how organic mercury in fish contributes to neurodevelopmental delays in children. The consensus among public health professionals is that women who are planning to have a baby, or who become pregnant, should avoid eating larger fish that are known to contain high levels of organic mercury. This is why the FDA issued a fish advisory in 2004, warning pregnant women against eating swordfish, albacore tuna, and other large fish species.[14]

Smaller fish, on the other hand, contain little organic mercury and are thought to benefit the pregnant woman and her developing fetus. The bottom line is that, if a pregnant woman eats the fish and shellfish listed on page 136, her child's risk of exposure to organic mercury appears to be extremely low. The child's crucial need for omega-3 outweighs the extremely low risk of organic mercury exposure associated with the consumption of these foods. Dietary DHA from appropriate fish, shellfish, and algae consumption is essential for proper brain development and will make a positive difference in the developing fetus and child,[18] especially in the case of children with autism and/or ADHD.[19,20,21]

Wild salmon—fresh or frozen, and cooked on your barbeque or in your oven—is your best bet. Salmon is very low in mercury and high in omega-3 fatty acids, according to Dr. Kate Mahaffey, a famous mercury researcher who was a principal author of the 1997 Mercury Study Report to Congress.[22] Figure 8.2 on page 138 is a graph she shared with me of her findings of organic methylmercury levels in different fish species.

As you can see, the black bar represents the organic methylmercury levels. The higher the black bar, the higher the organic mercury levels. Organic mercury levels are very high in tuna, sea bass, snap-

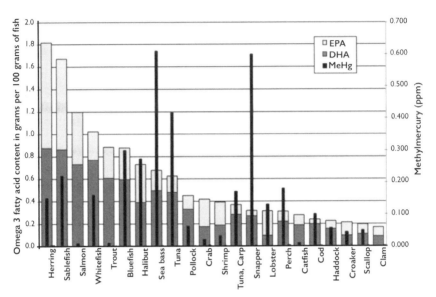

Figure 8.2. Comparing EPA, DHA, and organic methylmercury levels in various fish.

per, lobster, and perch. There is mercury in cod, so when you buy cod liver oil, make sure you buy the oil that was tested and certified "mercury-free." Swordfish and shark are not included in the chart, but both can have methylmercury levels of up to 1 ppm, according to the FDA.[23]

In addition to salmon, there are several other species that contain very low or no organic mercury, including crab, shrimp, catfish, clams, and trout. All of these smaller fish and shellfish are good dietary choices for increasing a child's omega-3 fatty acid intake levels.

One last significant concept is that if a child is zinc-deficient, you are not likely to see any improvement in his behavior or learning capacity, even if you boost his intake of omega-3 DHA. This is because zinc is needed by the body to utilize the omega-3 fatty acids that brain cells need to survive.[24] The two elements work hand in hand to keep brain cells healthy. Therefore, diets deficient in both zinc and omega-3 fatty acids contribute to the development of autism and ADHD in children.[16] It is so important for a child to eat a diet that is rich in *both* zinc and omega-3. Moreover, zinc is important for utilizing protein, as you will learn in the next section.

PROTEINS

Proteins are used by your body to transport sugar molecules and other nutrients into and out of your cells. Some proteins serve as antibodies in your immune system or hormones in your reproductive system. Other proteins work to make your muscles and bones strong. Proteins do the work required to keep your body healthy. The most important aspect of dietary protein is its role in contributing amino acids for the building of new proteins inside your body.[2] (See "The Molecular Structure of Protein" below for a more detailed explanation of amino acids.)

One very important type of protein that performs a wide range of functions in various cellular processes is the zinc finger protein. Zinc fingers are active in cell division and repair, protein production, turning genes on and off, metabolism, and communication systems.[25] Dietary zinc is essential to maintain the zinc balance in the body to facilitate gene expression, intracellular communication, bone growth, and the body's immune system.[26] It is important to incorporate foods in the diet that are high in both protein and zinc.

The Molecular Structure of Protein

Proteins are made up of amino acids, which are simply molecules containing the elements nitrogen (N), oxygen (O), carbon (C), and hydrogen (H). These molecules are then attached to a unique chemical "R group," which gives the protein its specific function. Amino acid molecules are the building blocks required by your body for building new proteins.

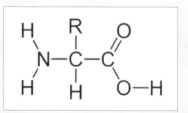

Figure 8.3. An amino acid molecule.

There are twenty different amino acid building blocks, each with a different "R group" that we know of, and thousands of different protein configurations that perform thousands of different functions.

Dietary Recommendations for Protein

Protein deficiency has been shown to adversely impact brain health, kidney function, and gut permeability.[2] In addition, inadequate protein intake may depress the immune system, leading to a higher risk of infections.[2] Table 8.1 below provides a list of foods high in both zinc and protein (listed from highest to lowest zinc content).[27]

Table 8.1. Foods Rich in Zinc and Protein

Zinc and Protein-Rich Food	Serving Size	Zinc Content (mg)	Protein Content (g)
Oysters, smoked, in olive oil	3 oz	74	14
Beef, chuck, lean, roast, all grades, fat trimmed, cooked	3 oz	8.73	22.6
King Crab, cooked	3 oz	6.48	16.5
Lamb, shoulder roast, arm, lean, fat trimmed, cooked	3 oz	6.21	21
Chicken, giblets, cooked	1 cup	6.13	38.8
Beans, cooked, plain	1 cup	5.79	12.1
Crab, canned	1 cup	5.43	24.1
Beef, ground, 85 percent lean, 15 percent fat, patty, cooked	3 oz	5.36	22
Turkey, meat, cooked, roasted	1 cup	4.34	52.1
Oat bran, raw	1 cup	2.92	16.3
Yogurt, plain, skim	8 oz	2.2	13
Mushrooms, shiitake, cooked, without salt	1 cup	1.93	2.26
Nuts, pine nuts, dried	1 oz	1.83	3.9

It makes sense that foods rich in protein would also be rich in zinc, given the role zinc finger plays in so many different protein functions. Table 8.1 does not list all protein- and zinc-rich foods, but lists the whole, unprocessed foods tested by the USDA and found to contain the highest amounts of zinc.[28] Notice the recommendation within the table for eating lean (low in fat) red meat (e.g., lamb and beef) and low-fat yogurt. The purpose of minimizing the intake of fat from these foods is to reduce saturated fats, which contribute to the development of heart disease. Appropriate protein intake is necessary for proper gene function throughout the human lifespan to sustain health. Unfortunately, appropriate protein intake in the U.S. is currently lacking, according to a few recent studies.

Current American Protein Dietary Pattern

A recent study conducted by scientists with no competing interests indicates American infants and children are not eating the appropriate amount of protein. In 2015, dietary intake data from the 2005–2012 United States National Health and Nutrition Examination Survey (NHANES) was analyzed by Australian scientists, led by Carley Grimes, who wanted to determine the food sources of energy and nutrients among U.S. infants and toddlers.[29] Such a study had not been conducted on this age group in the U.S. since 2002.[29] Grimes et al. found that two-thirds of U.S. infants between the ages of 0–11.9 months were not being breastfed.[29] Human breast milk is the most important source of protein for infants during their first year of life.[29]

Grimes et al. also found that U.S. toddlers' diets were lacking in iron and zinc because they were eating significantly more grain- and cereal-based foods and nutrient-poor processed meats instead of meats high in iron and zinc.[29] The scientists found the kinds of meat being eaten by the U.S. toddlers consisted primarily of processed, cured meat and poultry, which likely contributed to their excessive intakes of sodium and saturated fat.[29] Grimes et al. encouraged American families to switch from cold cuts, bacon, frankfurters, and sausages to non-processed, lean meats, which are high in zinc, iron, and potassium and low in sodium and saturated fat.[29] Such encouragement coming from uncompromised scientists outside of the U.S. who have analyzed what we eat is without precedence.

In an article published in 2015, U.S. military scientists reported their findings of a study of the protein intake of U.S. adults aged nineteen and older during the 2007–2010 period.[30] The military scientists analyzed the NHANES dietary intake data collected from 10,977 American adults.[30] They found animal and dairy protein sources accounted for two-thirds of total protein intake, while plant-based protein sources accounted for one-third.[30] The largest contributors to the total plant protein intake were grains, which were accounted for in the diet survey with the reported consumption of foods such as doughnuts, cakes, pies, biscuits, and bread.[30] The military scientists suggested that overconsumption of these foods likely diminishes the quality of the total protein intake because these foods are made of refined grains and likely contain added sugar.[30] Such composition results in a less protein-dense food with negative impacts on health.[30]

In another article, published in 2016, scientists reported that elderly Americans also are not meeting their recommended dietary allowance for protein.[31] The scientists, led by Beasley in New York City, studied the protein intake of 1,011 elderly men and women aged sixty to ninety-nine years.[31] They found that just 33 percent of women and 50 percent of men reported eating their recommended dietary allowance for protein.[31] The elderly citizens who ate at least 0.8 grams of protein per kilogram of body weight each day had less body fat.[31] Another study published in 2016 confirmed that a higher-protein diet is associated with less body fat and a lower risk of heart disease.[32]

From this brief review of recent studies, it does not seem to make a difference whether the protein is plant- or animal-based as long as the *quality* of the protein is good. Hopefully, you have learned that high-quality protein is low in both saturated fat and sodium; unprocessed; high in zinc, iron, or potassium; unrefined; and whole in nature. All of the foods listed in Table 8.1 on page 140 are excellent sources for plant- and animal-based protein. In the next section, you will learn a similar standard of quality applies to foods that provide your body with carbohydrates.

CARBOHYDRATES

Carbohydrates, or sugar chains, are a diverse family of molecules ranging in length and complexity. (See "The Molecular Structure of Carbohydrates" below.) Glucose and fructose are simple in form, whereas starch is more complex. These and other carbohydrates are found primarily in plant-based foods. Fruits, vegetables, potatoes, and whole grains are all rich sources of carbohydrates. When you eat these foods, they are broken down into the individual sugar molecules. Your body needs carbohydrates primarily for obtaining glucose to perform the work of cells. The oxygen in the air you breathe combines with the glucose in the carbohydrates you eat to

The Molecular Structure of Carbohydrates

Carbohydrates are, by definition, chains of sugar molecules. Each sugar molecule is made up of carbon (C), hydrogen (H), and oxygen (O) atoms. The arrangement of atoms for each type of sugar molecule is different. The number of carbon atoms in a simple sugar molecule can range from three to seven, depending on the type of sugar molecule.[7] Five and six carbon sugars form molecular rings. Different types of sugar rings can join together. For example, glucose and fructose can join together to form honey, sucrose (table sugar), or high fructose corn syrup (HFCS).[7] The following diagram shows the carbon rings of glucose and fructose joining together to form sucrose.

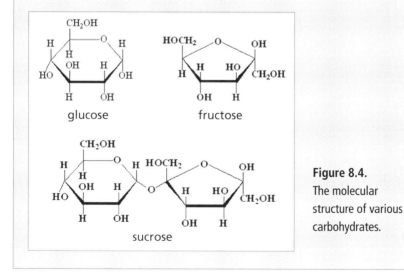

Figure 8.4.
The molecular structure of various carbohydrates.

produce the energy your cells need to conduct work.[7] If you did not have glucose in your blood, your cells would not be able to provide the energy needed for tissue repair.[7] Glucose also provides your cells with some of the raw material needed for making proteins, which your body needs in order to function.[7] In short, your body needs glucose. However, you should ensure that your dietary source of glucose is minimally processed.

For example, honey is made by honey bees and should undergo no processing before it reaches your grocery store. Table sugar, or sucrose, is made from the stems of sugarcane or the roots of sugar beets.[7] In Chapter 4, we discussed how HFCS is manufactured from corn using a variety of chemicals, including the inorganic mercury compound named *mercuric chloride.* Honey, sugar, and HFCS are carbohydrates commonly listed as food ingredients on food product labels. Of the three ingredients, honey should contain the fewest contaminants due to its natural origin. Honey produced by local farmers is your best choice for a natural sweetener. HFCS, on the other hand, needs to be avoided.

Your body does not need every type of carbohydrate you eat. The liver is strategically located above your gut,[7] and this is where unneeded or toxic carbohydrates end up. Unlike glucose, fructose is not needed by your body and is, in fact, considered a toxic substance.[33] It is converted to fat in the liver.[33] Having excess fat in the liver is, by definition, fatty liver disease. Your liver does its best to detoxify fructose, but excess consumption of high fructose-containing foods or ingredients (such as HFCS) can lead to nonalcoholic fatty liver disease, which is becoming more common in the U.S. population. (See "Fructose and Fatty Liver Disease in the U.S." below.)

Fructose and Fatty Liver Disease in the U.S.

Fatty liver disease not associated with alcohol consumption is called nonalcoholic fatty liver disease, or NAFLD for short. As with alcohol, excess fructose consumption may, over time, lead to cirrhosis (scarring of the liver) and functional impairment of the liver.[34,35,36,37]

Scientists recently conducted an analysis of the NHANES biomarker data collected from 11,674 Americans to determine the prevalence of NAFLD in the U.S. population.[38] The scientists studied the occurrence of the symptoms associated with NAFLD, including impaired fasting glucose/diabetes, high triglyceride levels, low high-density lipoprotein (HDL) levels, high blood pressure, and increased waist circumference.[38] They determined the prevalence of symptomatic NAFLD among the tested subjects was 18.2 percent.[38] Liver ultrasounds were also conducted to determine the prevalence of NAFLD in the subjects who did not yet show any metabolic symptoms.[38] The prevalence of asymptomatic NAFLD was 6.1 percent.[38] The results of this important study indicate that the total NAFLD prevalence in the American adult population is currently 24.3 percent—almost one-quarter of adults in the U.S. now have NAFLD!

NAFLD is becoming more common in obese children; this has been associated with dietary fructose intake.[39] In a recent clinical trial, scientists found that dietary fructose restriction improved the metabolic parameters in obese children at risk of NAFLD.[40] Specifically, with the fructose restriction, scientists observed significant reductions in blood pressure, triglyceride levels, and glucose levels of the American children under study.[40] This impressive outcome showed that improvements in diet alone can alleviate the metabolic symptoms associated with NAFLD.

NAFLD is a major cause of liver disease in the U.S.[41,42] NAFLD is the beginning stage of chronic liver disease, which ends in death if not successfully treated.[41,42] Between 1999 and 2013, the death rate from chronic liver disease and cirrhosis rose by 50 percent in white non-Hispanic Americans between the ages of 45–54.[42] This astounding finding was published in 2015 in the *Proceedings of the National Academy of Sciences*.[42] To prevent NAFLD, it is important to reduce the intake of high fructose-containing foods and ingredients and increase the intake of healthy carbohydrates, which will be discussed in the next section.

Dietary Recommendations for Carbohydrates

You've probably heard of low-carb diets; many weight loss programs and products are available on the market to encourage consumers to reduce their intake of carbohydrates. Contrary to popular belief, such diets will not lead to lasting and long-term weight loss. It is true that the quantity and *quality* of carbohydrate intake is associated with the risk of obesity and a number of chronic diseases to include type 2 diabetes, cancer, and heart disease.[43] If your carbohydrate intake primarily consists of refined grains, sugars, and beverages containing high fructose corn syrup, then you will significantly increase your risk of developing any one of these chronic diseases. What most consumers fail to understand is the fact that increased intake of whole vegetables, grains, fiber, and fruits will decrease your risk of obesity and chronic disease. There are essentially "good" carbs and "bad" carbs.[44] If you want to lose weight, then you must eliminate your intake of "bad" carbs (highly processed foods) and increase your intake of "good" carbs. Below are examples of each type of carb.[44]

Good Carbs

- Broccoli, cauliflower
- Brown rice, oats, quinoa, barley
- Green leafy vegetables (spinach, greens, Swiss chard)
- Legumes (beans)
- Nuts
- Plain yogurt, low-fat cheese
- Reduced fat (2%) milk
- Whole oranges, apples, other fruits and berries

Bad Carbs

- Alcohol
- Baked goods (bread, cookies, pies, cakes, crackers, pastries)
- Fruit juice
- Pizza
- Potato chips
- Potatoes, French fries
- Processed foods
- Sugar-sweetened beverages, soft drinks

The lists above show that whole foods are a good source of carbohydrates. They were generated, in part, from a paper published by a Harvard research team led by Dr. Dariush Mozaffarian.[44] Mozaffarian et al. followed 120,877 American men and women for many years to determine which dietary and lifestyle factors would lead to obesity.[44] At the beginning of the study, all of the men and women were free of chronic disease and were not obese.[44] The findings of the study were published in the *New England Journal of Medicine* in 2011.[44] Mozaffarian et al. found that consumption of processed foods (bad carbs) is independently and positively associated with long-term weight gain in the U.S.[44] This means that even if you exercise, you will gain weight if your diet consists primarily of bad carbs. Consumption of vegetables, nuts, fruits, and whole grains is associated with less weight gain, even when you eat larger portions.[44] Mozaffarian et al. also found that consumption of all liquids except milk and water is positively associated with weight gain.[44] A smaller study conducted in Canada found that a low-carbohydrate diet is associated with the development of obesity in healthy adults over time.[45] What this means is to prevent obesity, you need to eat a diet high in *good* carbs.

Good carbs contain the elements necessary for maintaining good health. We've talked about some of these important elements in previous chapters—calcium, phosphorus, magnesium, and methyl-donating nutrients. We've discussed the role of calcium and methyl-donating nutrients in gene function. Chapter 5 provides tables that list foods high in calcium and high in methyl-donating nutrients. A quick review of these tables will reveal that many of these foods also contain good carbs. The bottom line is that you want to avoid consuming bad carbs by reducing your intake of refined and processed foods containing sugars, corn sweeteners, vegetable oils, and other unhealthy food ingredients. These bad carbs have little or no nutritional value. When it comes to weight control and health, the type of carbohydrate matters more than the number of calories you eat. There is a difference between bad carbs and good carbs.

ADDITIONAL SUGGESTIONS

In addition to the all of the above recommendations regarding lipids, proteins, and carbohydrates, I would also suggest the following guidelines:

- Avoid all added sugars, including corn sweeteners.

- Avoid all products containing trans fat.

- Avoid eating fast food.

- Avoid eating hydrogenated or partially hydrogenated vegetable oils.

- Avoid eating processed foods.

- Buy frozen if you cannot find fresh.

- Buy organic to reduce your overall pesticide exposure whenever possible.

- Drink water with every meal and in between.

- Limit your intake of 100 percent juice to one small glass a day.

For more specific information on removing pesticides from produce that is not organic, see "How to Eliminate or Reduce Pesticide Exposures" below.

How to Reduce or Eliminate Produce Pesticide Exposures

Several studies have been conducted by U.S. government and university scientists to determine whether substituting organic fresh fruits and vegetables for corresponding conventional food items will reduce pesticide exposures.[46,47,48] The results of these studies indicate that switching to an organic diet will significantly reduce or even *eliminate* pesticide exposures, especially in young children.[46,47,48] Unfortunately, switching to an organic diet may be too expensive for some consumers.

If your wallet will not support your eating an organic diet, know that you can still reduce your pesticide exposures from conventionally grown produce. Rinsing your produce with tap water has been found to significantly reduce pesticide residues across all commodities.[49,50] I myself use the tap water rinsing method to decontaminate my conventional produce if I cannot buy organic. Chlorinated tap water is certainly less harmful than the pesticide residues found on conventionally grown fruits and vegetables. How do we know the tap water rinsing method works?

Scientists at the University of Connecticut initiated a research program in 1997 to examine the effect of tap water rinsing on reducing

FOOD ALLERGIES AND FAMILY HEALTH

Many families use caution when selecting their groceries because of a food allergy. Some people may have developed a food allergy from their diets and are unaware of it. The quality of life may be significantly impacted in people who suffer from food allergies or sensitivity to chemicals. Formula-fed infants, in particular, are especially at risk of developing a food or chemical allergy due to their undeveloped immune systems.[52] Individuals can become allergic to a variety of substances found in the food supply, such as cow's milk protein, wheat, proteins found in wheat, copper, and even mercury. Whether or not specific genes are turned on or off may play a role in the development of some of these allergies.[53,54,55] Some people have a genetic variation that makes them hypersensitive to mercury.[53] PON1 gene variation can make certain people hypersensitive to mercury or

---

pesticide residues in produce.[49,50] They also examined the effect of fruit and vegetable wash products and a one percent liquid detergent solution on pesticide residues in produce.[49,50] It turns out that the key factor in reducing the pesticide residues using the tap water rinsing method is that the produce must be held under running water and rubbed for at least thirty seconds.[49,50] In comparing their results, the scientists concluded that water rinsing with the mechanical rubbing action for thirty seconds is as effective as washing produce with a mild detergent or fruit and vegetable wash.[49,50]

The National Pesticide Information Center provides the following additional tips for reducing harmful pesticide exposures:[51]

- Discard outer layer of leafy vegetables (e.g., lettuce, spinach, chard).
- Do not soak or dunk produce.
- Eat a variety of fruits and vegetables to minimize exposure to a single pesticide.
- Grow your own garden.
- Peel fruits and vegetables whenever possible.
- Scrub firm fruits and vegetables (e.g., melons, potatoes, carrots).
- Wash all produce under running water, even the organic produce.

organophosphate pesticide residues.[53,56] In Chapter 7, we briefly discussed the most common allergens recognized by the U.S. government. Symptoms of allergy include those listed below:[57]

Symptoms of Food/Food Ingredient Allergy and/or Chemical Sensitivity

- Aggression

- Depression or lethargy, moodiness, crying, emotional sensitivity

- Difficulty reading (dyslexia) and writing (dysgraphia)

- Extreme silliness, unrestrained behavior

- Finger tapping, tics, tremors

- Hyperactivity, extreme talkativeness

- Hypersensitivity to odors, light, cold, pain, touch, sound

- Impulsivity

- Inattention, difficulty concentrating, forgetfulness

- Mental confusion

- Nervousness or inability to look others in the eye

- Tiredness, drowsiness, lack of energy

If you suspect that you or a member of your family has an allergy, please consult an appropriately trained specialist who can rule out suspected allergens. A diagnosis of food intolerance or allergy to suspected allergens may involve blood serum testing, skin-prick testing, food diary analysis, or placing the patient on an elimination diet.[58] A physician specializing in diagnosing and identifying allergies is an allergist or immunologist. Gastroenterologists (doctors who specialize in the digestive tract) are also particularly well-versed in food allergies.

If you eliminate harmful food ingredients and pesticide exposures from your family's diet, I think you will find that your family's health will improve. If you have a child with autism or ADHD, your child's behavior and ability to learn will most certainly improve over time, especially as the heavy metal levels decrease in his bloodstream when processed foods are removed from his diet.[59,60] This is what the science-based evidence that has been presented in this book tells us.

CONCLUSION

All people have genetic variations that make them more susceptible to adverse health outcomes, including the development of disease, when diet is poor. Allergies, cancer, Alzheimer's, autism, heart disease, ADHD, and type 2 diabetes are all examples of adverse health outcomes associated with poor diet. As we've learned in this book, the highly processed Standard American Diet (SAD) is deficient in key nutrients and ridden with toxic substance residues that may modify gene behavior, creating conditions for the development of disease. What you eat or don't eat is your body's only defense against the development of disease.

In this chapter, we've discussed the reason why we eat, which is to obtain the macromolecules our body needs to thrive. The quality of food you keep in your kitchen pantry and refrigerator will determine the quality of the lipids, proteins, and carbohydrates you eat in your diet. In this chapter, I've provided you with various lists and tables that list the best sources for obtaining each macromolecule; guidelines for a healthy diet; and a food pyramid to help you visualize the type and quantity of foods you need to eat. Hopefully, you will now have a better idea of how to create a healthy food environment at home.

Conclusion

In this book, you have learned about the various toxic substances that can be found in our food supply, how they get there, and their effects on consumers' health and well-being. You now may be wondering what, if anything, the federal government is doing to reduce these toxic substance exposures. Unfortunately, the government is not as focused on policies and education regarding this issue as it should be, partly because it is placing its attention on foodborne illnesses.

THE FOODBORNE ILLNESS FRENZY

There are many stakeholders involved in the food distribution system, and all have differing views on the safety of the food supply. Despite these differing views, the American food safety system is focused almost exclusively on reducing foodborne illnesses associated with exposures to infectious agents. Occurring several times a year, the U.S. government and the press are quick to report outbreaks associated with *Salmonella, E. coli,* or some other infectious agent. It is always important to warn the public if a product is contaminated with an infectious agent. To reduce the occurrence of such contaminants, the U.S. Congress passed the 2011 Food Safety Modernization Act (FSMA), which empowers FDA to further regulate food facilities and begin regulating farms to minimize foodborne disease outbreaks.

The FSMA requires food facilities to develop formal, written food safety plans to prevent, identify, and correct any issues likely to cause a foodborne illness, such as bacterial contamination on surfaces and in products.[1] The food safety plans must include preventive measures that incorporate process and sanitation controls and guidelines for recalling products if contaminants are found.[1] All actions taken under the food safety plan must be documented and presented to the FDA food police upon demand.[1]

The FSMA also requires farms making more than $25,000 a year from the sale of produce to comply with new sanitation regulations.[2] Specifically, water quality testing is now mandatory if the farm's water supply does not come from a chemically treated public water system.[3] Farmers must pay for the testing of their agricultural water to determine whether *E. coli* bacteria is present.[3] If *E. coli* is present, the farmers must take corrective action.[3] Farmers must also provide their farm workers with specific health and hygiene training to prevent the spread of infectious agents.[3]

All covered food facilities and farms are now required to register with the FDA and pay a $500 fee. Compliance with the new FSMA regulations is expected to cost food facilities and individual farmers several thousand dollars a year. Enforcement of the regulations by FDA food police and government contractors will cost millions of dollars a year, according to current budget estimates.[4] The focus of the unprecedented reach of the new regulations is to further prevent the spread of foodborne illness through improvements in sanitation.

With the FDA so focused on the prevention of foodborne illness, you are probably thinking the food supply must be very unsanitary. After all, foodborne disease outbreaks are widely publicized, as are the sanitation issues associated with them; the focus on these regulations must be warranted. Nothing could be further from the truth. I assure you the American food supply is extremely sanitary.

This book has provided information on the use of inorganic mercury and other toxic substance residues in food processing and manufacturing to ensure the timely death of every living organism finding its way into the food supply. While the system is not perfect, few people die each year of a foodborne illness associated with unsanitary conditions. We know this because the U.S. Centers for Disease Control (CDC) estimates the occurrence of foodborne illness—and deaths occurring from such illness—each year.[5] CDC scientists collect hard data to make their estimates. Recently, they conducted a study of hospitalizations in the U.S. that occurred between 2000 and 2008 and estimated that on average, 1,351 Americans die each year of a foodborne illness.[6] Of those deaths, CDC scientists determined twenty were due to *E. coli* and 378 were due to *Salmonella*.[6]

Over 1,300 deaths per year from foodborne illness might seem excessive, but this number is quite small when you consider the number of Americans who die each year from diseases associated with eating the Standard American Diet (SAD). Throughout this book, we've discussed all of the SAD factors—such as poor diet from eating highly processed foods, exposures to toxic substances via allowable pesticide and heavy metal residue levels, and the impact of these exposures on gene behavior—associated with the development of the Western diseases.

Table 1 compares average annual deaths from foodborne illness[6] to the most recent CDC mortality data for preventable diseases associated with poor diet and toxic substance exposures:[7]

Table 1. Annual Deaths from Foodborne Illnesses and SAD-Related Diseases

Cause of Death	Number of Deaths in the U.S. (2014)
Foodborne illness	1,351
Heart disease	614,348
Cerebrovascular disease	133,103
Alzheimer's disease	93,541
Diabetes mellitus	76,488
Chronic liver disease	38,170
Hypertension and hypertensive renal disease	30,221
Parkinson's disease	26,150

From the data in the table, it is clear to me—and I hope it is clear to you—what needs to be done. Food safety and public health policies need to focus on preventing the chronic diseases associated with poor diet and toxic substance exposures from the consumption of processed foods. The new and costly regulations released by FDA under FSMA will not significantly improve public health outcomes because they are focused primarily on reducing foodborne illness. On the contrary, hundreds of thousands of Americans will continue to die and suffer each year from the debilitating diseases caused by poor diet and co-exposures to the toxic substances in the food supply.

WHAT THE FDA CAN DO

As a health educator and former FDA researcher in the know, I suggest a new approach to improving American quality of life and health outcomes: At the federal level, FDA could require food manufacturers to test food products for the presence of inorganic mercury and other heavy metals at detectable levels. Manufacturers using food ingredients known or allowed to contain certain heavy metals could easily be required to test their products and provide warnings on food packaging to consumers on the presence or absence of heavy metal residues. Such labeling would help consumers make informed choices about the foods they buy. If FDA can require farmers making $25,000 a year from the sale of produce to test their agricultural waters for *E. coli*, surely FDA can require the billion-dollar food industry manufacturers to test their processed foods for inorganic mercury or other heavy metal residues. The U.S. Congress must act to pass legislation giving FDA this authority now!

Alternatively, the FDA could simply ban the use of food ingredients or processing aids known to contain heavy metals. There is precedence for FDA to act without Congressional authority. FDA has removed unhealthy food ingredients or substances from the food supply before, even in cases when the substance was previously considered safe and had GRAS status. For example, in 2013, FDA made the determination that artificial trans fat should be removed from the food supply.[8] FDA determined these partially hydrogenated oils (PHOs) are no longer considered generally recognized as safe (GRAS) for use in any human food.[8] These PHOs are commonly found in many processed foods and have been used by manufacturers to increase the shelf life and stability of foods since the 1950s.[8]

Why did the FDA decide to ban PHOs? Because "various studies have consistently linked *trans* fat consumption to heart disease."[8] Furthermore, "A 2002 report by the National Academy of Science's Institute of Medicine found a direct correlation between intake of *trans* fat and increased levels of low density lipoprotein (LDL) cholesterol, commonly referred to as 'bad' cholesterol, and, therefore, increased risk of heart disease."[8] The reasoning for the FDA ban is sound, in my opinion, but sadly there is more to the story that you should know.

Long ago, it was determined that PHOs in the oil and margarine industries contain inorganic mercury levels.[9] Furthermore, there is ample evidence to show that inorganic mercury is profoundly toxic to the heart.[10] Numerous studies describe the role inorganic mercury exposure plays in the development of heart disease. Many of these studies are described in the review article written by Azevedo et al. and published in 2012.[10] One toxic mechanism of inorganic mercury exposure known to produce atherosclerosis is increased levels of LDL.[10] Mercury levels are, in fact, predictors of the levels of LDL.[10] What this means is that the exact same reasoning FDA used to ban PHOs should now be used to ban the use of food ingredients and processing aids known to contain allowable levels of inorganic mercury.

At the federal level, FDA has the power to act now to remove one of the worst toxic substances in the food supply—inorganic mercury. In doing so, FDA could, on its own, pave the way for improvements in American quality of life and health outcomes. Inorganic mercury is associated with the development of all of the chronic diseases listed in Table 1 that lead to death, disability, and suffering.[10,11] Don't forget the results of the Fort Peck Community College study (described in Chapters 4 and 5), where my collaborators and I collected and analyzed data showing the direct correlation between inorganic mercury exposure (from the consumption of processed food) and the increased risk of developing type 2 diabetes.[11]

EDUCATION IS ESSENTIAL

At the state level, curriculum could be developed to teach nutrition and health education in community colleges and K–12 schools. This curriculum could incorporate the epigenetic role toxic substances in the food supply play in the development of disease. During our Fort Peck Community College study, we demonstrated how effective nutrition education can lead to improvements in diet and health outcomes in college students when dietary toxic substance exposures and epigenetics are topics of study.[11]

Guidelines for developing health education curricula for use in schools from pre-kindergarten to grade 12 are available from the CDC, although they do not address the role dietary toxic substance exposures play in the development of disease.[12] Particular attention should be given to CDC "guideline 5."[13] This guideline calls for health educators to provide students with the knowledge, attitudes, skills, and experiences needed for lifelong healthy eating.[13] Nutrition knowledge gained in youth from health education provided in schools can lay the foundation for the development of healthy eating habits that may last a lifetime. Since most disease conditions in the United States are preventable and related to what Americans eat,[14] current health education efforts that do not include nutrition as a component are going to be ineffective.

Currently, nutrition and cooking courses are not required for graduation from high school and certainly are not priority subjects in elementary and middle school. High school home economics courses have gone by the wayside. In the past, students would have learned about nutrition and honed their meal-planning skills in their home economics courses. By failing to incorporate nutrition and meal planning as instructional components in health education in K–12 schools, there will continue to be negative health outcomes, such as the growing obesity epidemic among American youth. Without nutrition and cooking education, youth may not develop an understanding of how dietary choices such as food preparation, meal frequency, and eating environment relate to the development of obesity and future disease conditions.[15] As young adults, they may then lack the prior knowledge they need to understand the requirements of a healthy diet and be unable to establish healthy eating habits for their own families.[16]

We know that unhealthy eating habits of young adult women play a role in creating a perinatal environment during and after pregnancy that creates conditions in their babies for neurodevelopmental delay, autism,[17,18] and attention deficit hyperactivity disorder (ADHD).[19] Prenatal nutrition education is therefore key to preventing these debilitating learning disorders that impact special education programs in our public schools. The availability of free nutrition education programs in the United States for pregnant women and new mothers varies depending on socioeconomic status. Women of lesser means with low income across the United States are provided with supplemental foods, nutrition education, and healthcare referrals through the Women, Infants and Children (WIC) program, funded by the U.S. Department of Agriculture.[20] WIC services are available for all low-income women, pregnant or postpartum, and to infants and children up to age five who are found to be at nutritional risk.[20] The states with the highest WIC participation have the lowest autism rates in the United States.[21] The nutrition education component of WIC surely plays a role in producing these lower rates of autism.

It is interesting to note that autism prevalence increases with increasing socioeconomic status.[22,23] The reason for this is presumably because families of greater means may not necessarily have the prior knowledge to understand the requirements of a healthy diet. Young adults across the U.S. are lacking a basic nutrition education, regardless of their socioeconomic status, because most K–12 schools are not providing this basic instruction. If the K–12 schools do not provide young people with nutrition education, then they may not have access to it, especially if their higher socioeconomic status prevents them from participating in the WIC nutrition education program.[20]

As we've learned throughout this book, what expectant mothers eat determines the quality of life and the health outcomes of their offspring. If the food a mother eats during pregnancy contains toxic substance residues and the quality of her diet is poor, then her baby's health will be at risk. It is so important to understand that what Mom eats while she is pregnant will not only determine her child's learning ability, but also how her child's genes will behave. Poor prenatal diet plays a role in the child's development of obesity and chronic diseases later in life. Once an infant enters the household, parent knowledge about nutrition will further impact the present and future health of the developing child, for better or worse. If the infant is prone to autism or ADHD, then feeding him formula contaminated with heavy metal residues will worsen his condition. As the infant becomes a child, feeding him the SAD of processed foods containing inorganic mercury and other heavy metals while offering little in the way of essential nutrients will likely result in the development of problematic behaviors and obesity. Remember that symptoms of autism and ADHD increase with exposures to heavy metals especially when important micronutrients such as zinc or calcium are lacking in the family diet.

Adults can't provide their children with a healthy family diet if they don't know how to plan and prepare meals that are free of toxic substance residues and contain the nutrients needed by the body. The success of the WIC program clearly shows that income alone is not the predictor of healthy eating habits or child health outcomes. Access to healthy foods and nutrition education that provides information about the quality of the food supply, safe meal planning, and preparation are key requirements in the adoption of healthy eating habits. Disease prevention cannot be accomplished without the adoption of healthy eating habits. Nutrition education in K–12 schools, colleges, and prenatal programs can pave the way to improvements in the American diet and health outcomes.

My collaborators and I have shown how effective nutrition education at the community college level can lead to improvements in diet that significantly reduce the risk of chronic disease in a lower-income population.[11] The same nutrition education has now been provided to you in this book. I hope the information helps you to make improvements in your diet that will enhance the quality of your life and reduce your risk of developing the chronic diseases associated with eating the SAD. I hope U.S. policymakers will also read this book.

NEXT STEPS

If you would like to take what you have learned in this book to the next level, an online tutorial is available on the Food Ingredient and Health Research Institute's website at foodingredient.info/safehealthy diettutor/syllabus.html. The tutorial was originally completed by parents of learning-disabled children as part of a clinical trial. After they had completed the tutorial, the participants took the information to heart and changed their diets to reduce intake of highly processed foods and increase their consumption of whole foods.[24]

This tutorial is composed of eight modules (one for each chapter of this book). By completing the activities in each module, you will gain a more comprehensive understanding of how environment and diet affect your genes and your health. During the tutorial, you will evaluate the foods that are currently in your kitchen and determine if they fit the criteria for safe foods. The tutorial will reinforce the information from this book about the Western dietary pattern and how you can improve upon it.[25]

CONCLUSION

With chronic disease conditions on the rise and healthcare costs skyrocketing, there is no time like the present to correct the policy problems in the food supply and education systems. Toxic substance residues can be eliminated from the food supply or food products can be tested and labeled if residues are present. Our policymakers have a role to play in ensuring the public has access to information about the contaminants in the food supply, healthy foods, and nutrition education. When the quality of food has the power to determine how our genes behave and whether or not we will succumb to disease or disability, we cannot ignore the contaminant problems that render much of our food supply unsafe to eat. As a society, we cannot afford to continue to live in an environment where our people are unsafe at any meal.

Resources

This section is to provide the reader with additional tools for ensuring a safe and healthy diet.

FREE WEB-BASED DIET TUTORIAL

Website: foodingredient.info/safehealthydiettutor/syllabus.html

The non-profit Food Ingredient and Health Research Institute (FIHRI) provides an online diet tutorial at no charge. The tutorial consists of eight modules of instruction. Each module is linked to a chapter in this book and includes clear learning objectives. Participants who complete the instruction are expected to achieve the following learning goals[1]:

1. Identify environmental and dietary factors that impact gene regulation leading to health or disease.

2. Examine Western dietary pattern over the last forty years and determine changes in the overall consumption of specific foods.

3. Survey kitchen cupboards, refrigerator, and freezer to identify food or food ingredients containing toxic substances that may impact gene function.

4. Recognize available resources for improving family diet and health.

5. Create a healthy food environment at home.

As you move through the modules, you will analyze components of the Western diet to better understand how environmental and dietary factors interact to protect your health or make you more susceptible to disease conditions. Topics include epigenetics, changes in U.S. dietary patterns over time, allowable toxic substance levels in food ingredients, regulatory role of FDA, conventional versus organic foods, micronutrients, and components of healthy diet.

RECOMMENDED VIDEOS

The Autism Revolution: Thinking about Environment and Food

Published by the Institute for Agriculture and Trade Policy on June 11, 2012.
Website: youtube.com/watch?v=mgAsDXgo5ao

This online seminar, led by Harvard pediatric neurologist Martha Herbert and independent researcher Renee Dufault, discusses the scientific discoveries about the relationship between toxic substance exposure and brain development in children.

Patterns of Health and Wellbeing 07: The Medicine of Food

Published by the Smithsonian Institute on April 29, 2014.
Website: youtube.com/watch?v=IwapwKitM0k

This symposium, led by Dr. Renee Dufault at the Smithsonian National Museum of the American Indian, details her research and collaboration with Native American communities to examine the link between cultural dietary changes and health.

Sugar: The Bitter Truth

Published by the University of California Television on July 30, 2009.
Website: youtube.com/watch?v=dBnniua6-oM

This lecture, led by pediatric endocrinologist Robert Lustig, details how sugar and fructose affect insulin levels and contribute to the obesity epidemic in America.

The Ghost in Your Genes

BBC Horizon documentary. First broadcast on November 3, 2005.
Website: dailymotion.com/video/x1f27b5_bbc-the-ghost-in-your-genes-2006xvid_tech

This documentary, brought to viewers by the BBC Horizons documentary series, introduces the study of epigenetics—how genes act in response to environment and life experience—and the researchers around the world who present evidence supporting this field.

LABORATORY RESEARCH

Agilent Technologies

Phone: (800) 227-9770
Email: agilent_inquiries@agilent.com
Website: agilent.com

Agilent Technologies is a company that provides laboratories worldwide with supplies and services, contributing to progressive scientific research. Agilent has published a report on exposomics, the study of how environmental exposures affect human biological functions. This report can be found at www.agilent .com/cs/library/brochures/5991-7004EN-Exposomics-Brochure.pdf.

Applied Isotope Technologies

Phone: (408) 472-2333
Email: info@sidms.com
Website: sidms.com

Applied Isotope Technologies creates technology that accurately measures and identifies specific elemental species in biological fluids and chemical compounds. Its technology is used in industrial and medical settings. Its innovations include screening tests that calculate body toxicant exposure. More information about the research that contributed to the development of these screening tests can be found at sidms.com/projects/exposomics.

ONLINE RESOURCES

Collaborative on Health and the Environment (CHE)

Phone: (360) 331-7904
Website: healthandenvironment.org

The CHE is a community of scientists, consumers, doctors, and other health-concerned citizens. Their mission is to evaluate health research and use it to promote health programs and policies. Their extensive overview of how the food we eat and how it is produced affect our health can be found at www.health andenvironment.org/what-we-know/environmental-contributors/food-and-agriculture-environment.

Environmental Protection Agency (EPA)
Certification of Laboratories for Drinking Water

Website: epa.gov/dwlabcert/contact-information-certification-programs-and-certified-laboratories-drinking-water

This section of the EPA website allows you to search for and contact laboratories in your state that conduct water quality testing for a reasonable price. For example, you can get your drinking water tested to determine lead or fluoride levels for about $15–$20.

Toxipedia

Phone: (206) 527-0926
Email: questions@toxipedia.org
Website: toxipedia.org

Toxipedia is an online encyclopedia of toxic substances. It was founded by Dr. Steven Gilbert. Pages are dedicated to ethical considerations, laws regarding toxic substances, associated health conditions, and other issues. It is a collaborative Wiki, meaning researchers, educators, and the general public are allowed to share knowledge and accurate information. It is a project of the non-profit Institute of Neurotoxicology and Neurological Disorders.

Centers for Disease Control and Prevention (CDC)

Phone: (800) 232-4636
Website: cdc.gov

The CDC is a government agency whose mission is to protect citizens from diseases and health threats. It tracks and analyzes how certain diseases spread across the nation or across the world and provides insight into possible solutions. Its article about the importance of a healthy food environment can be found at www.cdc.gov/healthyplaces/healthtopics/healthyfood_environment.htm.

Physicians for Social Responsibility (PSR)

Phone: (503) 274-2720
Website: psr.org

PSR's goal is to educate the public and campaign for government change in health and environmental policy. PSR wishes to promote peace in the quest for a healthy world. Its Oregon chapter has presented a Healthy Food Program that explains how food production and distribution can affect our health. It can be found here: www.psr.org/chapters/oregon/health-care-without-harm/healthy-food-program.html.

Clinical Epigenetics Article

Dufault, R, et al. "A macroepigenetic approach to identify factors responsible for the autism epidemic in the United States." *Clinical Epigenetics* 4(6): 2012.

Website: clinicalepigeneticsjournal.biomedcentral.com/articles/10.1186/ 1868-7083-4-6

In this article, which is available for the public online, my colleagues and I calculated the increase in the number of autistic children needing special education services between 2005 and 2010. We examined differences in diet and toxic substance exposure in two geographical populations to determine the extent of gene-environment interactions' effect on pervasive developmental disorders.

References

PREFACE

1. Dufault, R., Berg, Z., Crider, R., Schnoll R., Wetsit, L., Two Bulls, W., Gilbert, S., Kingston, S., Wolle, M., Rahman, M., & Laks, D. (2015). Blood inorganic mercury is directly associated with glucose levels in the human population and may be linked to processed food intake. *Integrative Molecular Medicine,* 2(3), 166-179. Retrieved from http://oatext.com/pdf/IMM-2-134.pdf

2. Goldman, L.R., Shannon, M.W., & Committee on Environmental Health. (2001). Technical report: mercury in the environment: implications for pediatricians. *Pediatrics,* 108, 197-205. Retrieved from http://pediatrics.aappublications.org/content/108/1/197.full.pdf

3. Schonwald, A. (2008). ADHD and food additives revisited. *AAP Grand Rounds,* 19;17. Retrieved from www.feingold.org/Research/PDFstudies/AAP08.pdf

4. Dufault, R., LeBlanc, B., Schnoll, R., Cornett, C., Schweitzer, L., Wallinga, D., Hightower, J., Patrick, L., & Lukiw, W.J. (2009). Mercury from chlor-alkali plants: measured concentrations in food product sugar. *Environmental Health,* 8:2. Retrieved from www.ehjournal.net/content/8/1/2

5. Rideout, K. (2010). Comment on the paper by Dufault et al.: Mercury in foods containing high fructose corn syrup in Canada. *Environmental Health,* 8:2. Retrieved from www.ehjournal.net/content/8/1/2/comments#418684.

6. Hilbeck, A., Binimelis, R., Defarge, N., Steinbrecher, R., Szekacs, A., Wickson, F., Antoniou, M., Bereano, P.L., Clark, E.A., Hansen, M., Novotny, E., Heinemann, J., Meyer, H., Shiva, V., & Wynne, B. (2015). No scientific consensus on GMO safety. *Environmental Sciences Europe,* 27:4. Retrieved from www.ensser.org/media/0115/

7. Karlsson, M. (2010). The precautionary principle in EU and US chemicals policy: a comparison of industrial chemicals legislation. In J. Eriksson, M. Gilek, & C. Rudén, (Eds.), *Regulating chemical risks* (pp. 239-265). Netherlands:Springer

8. Food Standards Agency. (2012). *Food colours and hyperactivity.* Retrieved from www.food.gov.uk/science/additives/foodcolours

9. McCann, D., Barrett, A., Cooper, A., Crumpler, D., Dalen, L., Grimshaw, K., Kitchin, E., Lok, K., Porteus, L., Prince, E., Sonuga-Barke, E., Warner, J., & Stevenson, J. (2007). Food

additives and hyperactive behavior in 3-year-old and 8/9-year-old children in the community: a randomized, double-blinded placebo-controlled trial. *Lancet* 2007, 370(9598), 1560-1567. www.feingold.org/Research/PDFstudies/Stevenson2007.pdf

10. Stevenson, J., Buitelaar, J. Cortese, S., et al. (2014). Research review: the role of diet in the treatment of attention-deficit/hyperactivity disorder—an appraisal of the evidence on efficacy and recommendations on the design of future studies. *Journal of Child Psychology and Psychiatry,* 55(5):416-427.

11. Nigg, J.T., Holton, K. (2014). Restriction and elimination diets in ADHD treatment. *Child Adolescent and Psychiatry Clinics of North America,* 23(4):937-953. Retrieved from www.ncbi.nlm.nih.gov/pmc/articles/PMC4322780/pdf/nihms660138.pdf

12. Dufault, R., Lukiw, W.J., Crider, R., Schnoll, R., Wallinga, D., & Deth, R. (2012). A macroepigenetic approach to identify the factors responsible for the autism epidemic in the United States. *Clinical Epigenetics,* 4:6. Retrieved from www.clinicalepigeneticsjournal .com/content/4/1/6

13. Dufault, R., Schnoll, R., Lukiw, W.J., LeBlanc, B., Cornett, C., Patrick, L., Wallinga, D., Gilbert, S.G., & Crider, R. (2009). Mercury exposure, nutritional deficiencies and metabolic disruptions may affect learning in children. *Behavioral and Brain Functions,* 5:44. Retrieved from www.behavioralandbrainfunctions.com/content/5/1/44

INTRODUCTION

1. Dufault, R., Abelquist, E., Crooks, S., Demers, D., DiBerardinis, L., Franklin, T., Horowitz, M., Petullo, C., & Sturchio, G. (2000). Reducing environmental risk associated with laboratory decommissioning and property transfer. Environmental Health Perspectives, 108(Supple 6), 1015-1022. Retrieved from www.ncbi.nlm.nih.gov/pmc/articles/ PMC1240234/pdf/ehp108s-001015.pdf or www.ensser.org/media/0115/

2. National Emission Standards for Hazardous Air Pollutants: Mercury Emissions from Mercury Cell Chlor-Alkali Plants, 76 Fed. Reg. 13852 (proposed Mar.14, 2011) (to be codified at 40 CFR Part 63). Retrieved from www.gpo.gov/fdsys/pkg/FR-2011-03-14/pdf/ 2011-5530.pdf

3. Luebke, P.W. (2004, May 6). E-mail correspondence regarding mercury levels found by Vulcan Chemical in their chemical products. Department of Natural Resources, Wisconsin.

4. Goldman, L.R., Shannon, M.W., & Committee on Environmental Health. (2001). Technical report: mercury in the environment: implications for pediatricians. Pediatrics, 108, 197-205. Retrieved from http://pediatrics.aappublications.org/content/108/1/197.full.pdf

5. United States Department of Agriculture. (2016). Food availability (per capita) data system. Retrieved from www.ers.usda.gov/data-products/food-availability-per-capita-data-system/

6. Dungan, A. (2004, May 13). E-mail correspondence regarding allowable mercury and lead levels in food grade mercury cell chlor-alkali chemicals according to regulations published in food chemicals codex: chlorine, sodium hydroxide, potassium hydroxide and hydrochloric acid. Chlorine Institute, Virginia.

7. US Pharmacopeial Convention. (2013). Food chemicals codex. Retrieved from www.usp.org/store/products-services/food-chemicals-codex-fcc

8. US Pharmacopeial Convention. (2013). About USP. Retrieved from www.usp.org/about-usp

9. Hightower, J.M. (2009). Diagnosis: mercury. Washington, DC: Island Press.

10. Environmental Protection Agency. (1971). Mercurial pesticides, man, and the environment. Available online via EPA National Service Center for Environmental Publications (NSCEP).

11. Corn Refiners Association. (2014). Why use HFCS? Retrieved from www.cornnaturally.com/Economics-of-HFCS/Why-Use-HFCS.aspx

12. National Institute of Standards and Technology, Chemical Science and Technology Laboratory. (2005). Measurement of organomercury and total mercury in corn syrup. (839.01-05-209).

13. Food Ingredient and Health Research Institute. (2014). What and who we are. Retrieved from www.foodingredient.info/whatandwhoweare.html

14. Food Ingredient and Health Research Institute. (2014). Our executive director. Retrieved from www.foodingredient.info/supporters/foundingdirector.html

CHAPTER 1

1. United States Food and Drug Administration. (2007). *Medicines in my home: caffeine and your body.* Retrieved from www.fda.gov/downloads/Drugs/ResourcesForYou/Consumers/BuyingUsingMedicineSafely/UnderstandingOver-the-CounterMedicines/UCM200805.pdf

2. United States Food and Drug Administration. (2016). *Why isn't the amount of caffeine a product contains required on a food label?* Retrieved from www.fda.gov/AboutFDA/Transparency/Basics/ucm194317.htm

3. Musgrave, I.F., Farrington, R.L., Hoban, C., & Byard, R.W. (2016). Caffeine toxicity in forensic practice: possible effects and under-appreciated sources. *Forensic Science, Medicine, & Pathology,* 12(3):299-303.

4. Przybilla, B., & Rueff, F. (2012). Insect stings. *Deutsches Arzteblatt International,* 109(13):238-248. Retrieved from www.ncbi.nlm.nih.gov/pmc/articles/PMC3334720/pdf/Dtsch_Arztebl_Int-109-0238.pdf

5. United States Food and Drug Administration. (2013). *FDA to investigate added caffeine.* Retrieved from www.fda.gov/ForConsumers/ConsumerUpdates/ucm350570.htm

6. United States Food and Drug Administration. (1978). Select committee on GRAS substances (SCOGS) opinion caffeine. Retrieved from www.fda.gov/Food/IngredientsPackagingLabeling/GRAS/SCOGS/ucm256650.htm

7. Tchounwou, P.B., Yedjou, C.G., Patiolla, A.K., & Sutton, D.J. (2012). Heavy metals toxicity and the environment. *EXS,* 101:133-164. Retrieved from www.ncbi.nlm.nih.gov/pmc/articles/PMC4144270/pdf/nihms414261.pdf

8. United States Environmental Protection Agency. (2011). *Questions and answers on fluoride.* Retrieved from www.epa.gov/sites/production/files/2015-10/documents/2011_fluoride_questionsanswers.pdf

9. Centers for Disease Control and Prevention. (2015). *Community water fluoridation.* Retrieved from www.cdc.gov/fluoridation/faqs/#fluoride3

10. Choi, A.L., Sun, G., Zhang, Y., & Grandjean, P. (2012). Developmental fluoride neurotoxicity: a systematic review and meta-analysis. *Environmental Health Perspectives,* 120:1362-1368. Retrieved from www.ncbi.nlm.nih.gov/pmc/articles/PMC3491930/pdf/ehp.1104912.pdf

11. Zeng, H., Shu, W., Chen, J., Liu, L., Wang, D., Fu, W., Wang, L., Luo, J., Zhang, L., Yan, Y., Qui, Z., & Huang, Y. (2014). Experimental comparison of the reproductive outcomes and early development of the offspring of rats given five common types of drinking water. *PLOS ONE,* 9(10):e108955. Retrieved from www.ncbi.nlm.nih.gov/pmc/articles/PMC4184831/pdf/pone.0108955.pdf

12. Sauerheber, R. (2013). Physiologic conditions affect toxicity of ingested industrial fluoride. *Journal of Environmental and Public Health.* Retrieved from www.ncbi.nlm.nih.gov/pmc/articles/PMC3690253/pdf/JEPH2013-439490.pdf

13. Dufault, R., LeBlanc, B., Schnoll, R., Cornett, C., Schweitzer, L., Wallinga, D., Hightower, J., Patrick, L., & Lukiw, W.J. (2009). Mercury from chlor-alkali plants: measured concentrations in food product sugar. *Environmental Health,* 8:2. Retrieved from www.ehjournal.net/content/8/1/2

14. Dufault, R., Schnoll, R., Lukiw, W.J., LeBlanc, B., Cornett, C., Patrick, L., Wallinga, D., Gilbert, S.G., & Crider, R. (2009). Mercury exposure, nutritional deficiencies and metabolic disruptions may affect learning in children. *Behavioral and Brain Functions,* 5:44. Retrieved from www.ncbi.nlm.nih.gov/pmc/articles/PMC2773803/#!po=76.0417

15. Islam, M.S., Ahmed, M.K., & Habibullah-Al-Mamun, M. (2014). Heavy metals in cereals and pulses: health implications in Bangladesh. *J Agric Food Chem,* 62(44):10828-10835.

16. Hsu, W.H., Jiang, S.J., & Sahayam, A.C. (2013). Determination of Cu, As, Hg, and Pb in vegetable oils by electrothermal vaporization inductively coupled plasma mass spectrometry with palladium nanoparticles as modifier. *Talanta,* 117, 268-272.

17. United States Environmental Protection Agency. (2016). *Chemical contaminant rules.* Retrieved from www.epa.gov/dwreginfo/chemical-contaminant-rules

18. Giblert-Diamond, D., Cottingham, K.L., Gruber, J.F., et al. (2011). Rice consumption contributes to arsenic exposure in US women. *PNAS,* 108(51):20656-20660. Retrieved from www.pnas.org/content/108/51/20656.full.pdf

19. Henn, B.C., Ettinger, A.S., Hopkins, M.R., et al. (2016). Prenatal arsenic exposure and birth outcomes among a population residing near a mining-related superfund site. *Environmental Health Perspectives,* DOI:10.1289/ehp.1510070. Retrieved from http://ehp.niehs.nih.gov/wp-content/uploads/advpub/2016/2/ehp.1510070.acco.pdf

20. National Institute of Health, U.S. Library of Medicine. (2016). *Cadmium.* https://toxtown.nlm.nih.gov/text_version/chemicals.php?id=63

21. Centers for Disease Control. (2013). *Cadmium toxicity: what diseases are associated with chronic exposure to cadmium?* www.atsdr.cdc.gov/csem/csem.asp?csem=6&po=12

22. Centers for Disease Control. (2013). *Cadmium toxicity: what are the U.S. standards for cadmium exposure?* Retrieved from www.atsdr.cdc.gov/csem/csem.asp?csem=6&po=7

23. Food and Agriculture Organization. (2007). *Carrageenan monograph.* Retrieved from www.fao.org/ag/agn/jecfa-additives/specs/monograph4/additive-117-m4.pdf

24. Centers for Disease Control. (2013). *Cadmium toxicity: what is the biological fate of cadmium in the body?*www.atsdr.cdc.gov/csem/csem.asp?csem=6&po=9

25. Jin, X., Tian, X., Liu, Z., et al. (2016). Maternal exposure to arsenic and cadmium and the risk of congenital heart defects in offspring. *Reproductive Toxicology,* 59:109-116.

26. Bellinger, D.C. (2016). Lead contamination in Flint—an abject failure to protect public health. New England Journal of Medicine, 374(12):1101-1103. Retrieved from www.nejm.org/doi/pdf/10.1056/NEJMp1601013

27. Kuehn, B. M. (2016). Pediatrician sees long road ahead for Flint after lead poisoning crisis. *Journal of the American Medical Association,* 315(10):967.

28. United States Environmental Protection Agency. (2016). *Table of regulated drinking water contaminants.* Retrieved from www.epa.gov/ground-water-and-drinking-water/table-regulated-drinking-water-contaminants

29. Rodriguez, E.G., Bellinger, D.C., Valeri, L., Hasan, M.O.S.I., Quamruzzaman, Q., Golam, M., Kile, M.L., Christiani, D.C., Wright, R.O., & Mazumdar, M. (2016). Neurode-velopmental outcomes among 2-to 3-year-old children in Bangladesh with elevated blood lead and exposure to arsenic and manganese in drinking water. *Environmental Health,* 15:44. Retrieved from www.ncbi.nlm.nih.gov/pmc/articles/PMC4788832/pdf/12940 _2016_Article_127.pdf

30. Grashow, R., Sparrow, D., Hu, H., & Weisskopf, M.G. (2015). Cumulative lead exposure is associated with reduced olfactory recognition performance in elderly men: the norma-tive aging study. *Neurotoxicology,* 49:158-164.

31. Joint FAO/WHO Expert Committee on Food Additives. (2002). *Limit test for heavy metals in food additive specifications: explanatory note.* Retrieved from www.fao.org/filead-min/templates/agns/pdf/jecfa/2002-09-10_Explanatory_note_Heavy_Metals.pdf

32. Institute of Medicine. (2003). *Food Chemicals Codex* 5th edition. Washington DC: National Academies Press; 2003.

33. World Health Organization.(2005). *Evaluation of certain food additives.* Retrieved from http://whqlibdoc.who.int/trs/WHO_TRS_928.pdf

34. United States Code of Federal Regulations. (2014). *Hydrochloric acid.* Retrieved from www.accessdata.fda.gov/scripts/cdrh/cfdocs/cfcfr/CFRSearch.cfm?fr=182.1057

35. Food and Agricultural Organization of the United Nations. (2006). *Chorine monograph.* Retrieved from www.fao.org/ag/agn/jecfa-additives/specs/Monograph1/Additive-126 .pdf

36. Dufault, R., Berg, Z., Crider, R., Schnoll R., Wetsit, L., Two Bulls, W., Gilbert, S., Kingston, S., Wolle, M., Rahman, M., & Laks, D. (2015). Blood inorganic mercury is directly associated with glucose levels in the human population and may be linked to processed food intake. *Integrative Molecular Medicine,* 2(3), 166-179. Retrieved from http://oatext.com/pdf/IMM-2-134.pdf

37. Laks, D.R. (2009). Assessment of chronic mercury exposure in the U.S. population, national health and nutrition examination survey, 1999-2006. *Biometals,* 22(6), 1103-14.

38. Dufault, R., Lukiw, W.J., Crider, R., Schnoll, R., Wallinga, D., & Deth, R. (2012). A macroepigenetic approach to identify the factors responsible for the autism epidemic in the United States. *Clinical Epigenetics,* 4:6. Retrieved from www.clinicalepigenetics journal.com/content/4/1/6

39. Food and Agricultural Organization of the United Nations. (2004). *Compendium of food additive specifications.* Retrieved from ftp://ftp.fao.org/es/esn/jecfa/addendum_12.pdf

40. United States Code of Federal Regulations. (2016). *Title 21, part 137: cereal flours and related products.* www.accessdata.fda.gov/scripts/cdrh/cfdocs/cfcfr/cfrsearch.cfm?fr=137.200

41. United States Food and Drug Administration. (1979). *Select committee on GRAS substances opinion: hydrochloric acid.* Retrieved from www.fda.gov/Food/IngredientsPackagingLabeling/GRAS/SCOGS/ucm260426.htm

42. European Feed Ingredients Safety Certification. (2013). *Sector reference document on the manufacturing of safe feed materials from oilseed crushing and vegetable oil refining.* www.efisc.eu/data/1377527038FEDIOL%20-%20version%203.0%20-%20Sector%20ref%20doc%20on%20oilseed%20crushing%20and%20veg%20oil%20refining%20version%203.0.pdf

43. United States Department of Agriculture. (2015). *Food availability per capita data system.* Retrieved from www.ers.usda.gov/data-products/food-availability-%28per-capita%29-data-system.aspx#.Ud3WT3-kBTY

44. Labtestsonline.org. (2016). *Cholinesterase.* Retrieved from https://labtestsonline.org/understanding/analytes/cholinesterase/

45. Lionetto, M.G., Caricato, R., Calisis, A., Giordano, M.E., & Schettino, T. (2013). Acetylcholinesterase as a biomarker in environmental and occupational medicine: new insights and future perspectives. *Biomedical Research International,* 321213. Retrieved from www.ncbi.nlm.nih.gov/pmc/articles/PMC3727120/pdf/BMRI2013-321213.pdf

46. The Human Exposome Project. (2016). *International exposome research projects.* Retrieved from http://humanexposomeproject.com/international-exposome-research-centers/

47. Vrijheid, M., Slama, R., Robinson, O., et al. (2014). The human early-life exposome (HELIX): project rationale and design. *Environmental Health Perspectives,* 122:534-544. Retrieved from http://ehp.niehs.nih.gov/wp-content/uploads/122/6/ehp.1307204.pdf

48. HERCULES Exposome Research Center. (2016). *Overview.* Retrieved from http://emoryhercules.com/about/overview/

49. HERCULES Exposome Research Center. (2016). *Research highlights.* Retrieved from http://emoryhercules.com/center-research/research-highlights/

50. United States Environmental Protection Agency. (2000). *Risk characterization handbook.* Retrieved from www.epa.gov/sites/production/files/2015-10/documents/osp_risk_characterization_handbook_2000.pdf

CHAPTER 2

Recommended Video

Holt, S., & Paterson, N. (2006). *Ghost in your genes.* [DVD]. Available for purchase from http://teacher.shop.pbs.org/product/index.jsp?productId=2916431

References

1. Public Broadcasting Service. (2007). *Epigenetics.* Retrieved from www.pbs.org/wgbh/nova/body/epigenetics.html

2. The Tech Museum of Innovation. (2013). *What is a gene?*http://genetics.thetech.org/about-genetics/what-gene

3. National Library of Medicine, National Institutes of Health. (2014). *What is the epigenome?*Retrieved from http://ghr.nlm.nih.gov/handbook/howgeneswork/epigenome

4. Volkmar, F.R., Klin, A., Schultz, R., Bronen, R., Marans, W.D., Sparrow, S., & Cohen, D.J. (1996). Asperger's syndrome. *J Am Acad Child Adolesc Psychiatry*, 35(1), 118-123.

5. Baron-Cohen, S., Ring, H., Chitnis, X., Wheelwright, S., Gregory, L., Williams, S., Brammer, M., & Bullmore, E. (2006). fMRI of parents of children with asperger syndrome: a pilot study. *Brain Cogn*, 61(1), 122-130.

6. Mohammadi, M.R., Zarafshan, H., & Ghasempour, S. (2012). Broader autism phenotype in Iranian parents of children with autism spectrum disorders vs normal children. *Iran J Psychiatry*, 7(4), 157-163. Retrieved from www.ncbi.nlm.nih.gov/pmc/articles/PMC3570573

7. Bradstreet, J.J., Smith, S., Baral, M., & Rossignol, D.A. (2010). Biomarker-guided interventions of clinically relevant conditions associated with autism spectrum orders and attention deficit hyperactivity disorder. *Altern Med Rev*, 15(1), 15-32. Retrieved from www.altmedrev.com/publications/15/1/15.pdf

8. Melnyk, S., Fuchs, G.J., Schultz, E., Lopez, M., Kahler, S.G., Fussell, J.J., Bellando, J., Pavliv, O., Rose, S., Seidel, L., Gaylor, D.W., & James, S. J. (2012). Metabolic imbalance associated with methylation dysregulation and oxidative damage in children with autism. *J Autism Dev Disord*, 42(3), 367-377. Retrieved from www.ncbi.nlm.nih.gov/pmc/articles/PMC3342663/

9. Frye, R.E., Melnyk, S., Fuchs, G., Reid, T., Jernigan, S., Pavliv, O., Hubanks, A., Gaylor, D.W., Walters, L., & James, S.J. (2013). Effectiveness of methylcobalamin and folinic acid treatment on adaptive behavior in children with autistic disorder is related to glutathione redox status. *Autism Res Treat*, epub: 609705. Retrieved from www.hindawi.com/journals/aurt/2013/609705/

10. Niculescu, M.D., Zeisel, S. H. (2002). Diet, methyl donors and DNA methylation: interactions between dietary folate, methionine, and choline. *J Nutr*, 132, 2333S-2335S. Retrieved from http://jn.nutrition.org/content/132/8/2333S.full

11. University of Utah. (2014). *Nutrition and the epigenome.* Retrieved from http://learn.genetics.utah.edu/content/epigenetics/nutrition/

12. Crider, K.S., Yang, T.P., Berry, R.J., & Bailey, L.B. (2012). Folate and DNA methylation: a review of molecular mechanisms and the evidence for folate's role. *Advances in Nutrition*, 3, 21-38. Retrieved from http://advances.nutrition.org/content/3/1/21.full.pdf+html

13. James, S.J., Melnyk, S., Jernigan, S., Hubanks, A., Rose, S., & Gaylor, D.W. (2008). Abnormal transmethylation/transsulfuration metabolism and DNA hypomethylation among parents of children with autism. *J Autism Dev Disord*, 38(10), 1966-1975. Retrieved from www.ncbi.nlm.nih.gov/pmc/articles/PMC2584168/

14. Kim, G.H., Ryan, J.J., Archer, S.L. (2013). The role of redox signaling in epigenetics and cardiovascular disease. *Antioxid Redox Signal*, 18(15), 1920-1936. Retrieved from www.ncbi.nlm.nih.gov/pmc/articles/PMC3624767/

15. Luttmer, R, Spijkerman, A.M., Kok, R.M., Jakobs, C., Blom, H.J., Serne, E.H., Dekker, J.

& M., Smulders, Y.M. (2013). Metabolic syndrome components are associated with DNA hypomethylation. *Obes Res Clin Pract,* 7(2), e106-e115.

16. Zawla, N.H., Lahiri, D.K., Cardozo-Pelaez, F. (2009). Epigenetics, oxidative stress and Alzheimer's disease. *Free Radical Biology and Medicine,* 46(9):1241-1249. Retrieved from www.ncbi.nlm.nih.gov/pmc/articles/PMC2673453/pdf/nihms99941.pdf

17. Hossein-nezhad, A.. Spira, A., & Holick, M.F. (2013). Influence of vitamin D status and vitamin D3 supplementation on genome wide expression of white blood cells: a random-ized double-blind clinical trial. *PLOS One,* 8, 3, e58725. Retrieved from www.ncbi .nlm.nih.gov/pmc/articles/PMC3604145/

18. National Library of Medicine, National Institutes of Health. (2014). *BDNF.* Retrieved from http://ghr.nlm.nih.gov/gene/BDNF

19. Zheng, F., Zhou, X., Moon, C., & Wang, H. (2012). Regulation of brain-derived neu-rotrophic factor expression in neurons. *Int J Physiol Pathophysiol Pharmacol,* 4(4), 188-200. Retrieved from www.ncbi.nlm.nih.gov/pmc/articles/PMC3544221/

20. Taurines, R., Segura, M., Schecklmann, M., Albantakis, L., Grunblatt, E., Walitza, S., Jans, T., Lyttwin, B., Haberhausen, M., Theisen, F.M., Martin, B., Briegel, W., Thomas, J., Schwenck, C., Romanos, M., & Gerlach, M. (2014). Altered peripheral BDNF mRNA expression and BDNF protein concentrations in blood of children and adolescents with autism spectrum disorder. *J Neural Transm,* 121(9), 1117-1128.

21. Graf-Myles, J., Farmer, C., Thurm, A., Royster, C., Kahn, P., Soskey, L., Rothschild, L., & Swedo, S. (2013). Dietary adequacy of children with autism compared with controls and the impact of restricted diet. *J Dev Behav Pediatr,* 34(7), 449-459. www.ncbi.nlm.nih.gov/pmc/articles/PMC3819433/

22. Buchman, A.S., Yu, L., Boyle, P.A., Schneider, J.A., De Jager, P.L., & Bennett, D.A. (2016). Higher brain BDNF gene expression is associated with slower cognitive decline in older adults. *Neurology,* 86(8):735-741.

23. Otsuka, M. (2015). Cognitive function and calcium. Intake of calcium and dementia. *Clinical Calcium,* 25(2):195-200.

24. Ozawa, M., Ninomiya, T., Ohara, T. et al. (2012). Self-reported dietary intake of potas-sium, calcium, and magnesium and risk of dementia in Japanese: the Hisayama Study. *Journal of American Geriatrics Society,* 60(8):1515-1520.

25. Wilson, R.S., Krueger, K.R., Boyle, P.A., Bennett, D.A. (2011). Loss of basic lexical knowledge in old age. *Journal of Neurology, Neurosurgery & Psychiatry,* 82(4):369-372. Retrieved from www.ncbi.nlm.nih.gov/pmc/articles/PMC3033766/pdf/nihms243469.pdf

26. Duverne, S., Lemaire, P., & Michel, B.F. (2003). Alzheimer's disease disrupts arithmetic fact retrieval processes but not arithmetic strategy selection. *Brain Cognition,* 52(3):302-318.

27. Machria, M., Hassan, M.S., Blackhurst, D., Erasmus, R.T., Matsha, T.E. (2012). The growing importance of PON1 in cardiovascular heath: a review. *J Cardiovasc Med (Hager-stown),* 13(7), 443-453.

28. Dufault, R., Lukiw, W.J., Crider, R., Schnoll, R., Wallinga, D., & Deth, R. (2012). A macroepigenetic approach to identify the factors responsible for the autism epidemic in the United States. *Clinical Epigenetics,* 4:6. Retrieved from www.clinicalepigeneticsjournal .com/content/4/1/6

29. United States Department of Agriculture. (2014). *Pesticide data program.* Retrieved from www.ams.usda.gov/AMSv1.0/ams.fetchTemplateData.do?template=TemplateC&navID=PesticideDataProgram&rightNav1=PesticideDataProgram&topNav=&leftNav=Science-andLaboratories&page=PesticideDataProgram&resultType

30. Costa, L.G., Giordano, G., & Furlong, C.E. (2011). Pharmacological and dietary modulators of paraoxonase 1 (PON1) activity and expression: the hunt goes on. *Biocheml Pharmacol, 81,* 337-344. Retrieved from www.ncbi.nlm.nih.gov/pmc/articles/PMC3077125/

31. Pasca, S.P., Dronca, E., Nemes, B., Kaucsar, T., Endreffy, E., Iftene, F., Benga, I., Cornean, R., & Dronca, M. (2010). Paraoxonase 1 activities and polymorphisms in autism spectrum disorders. *J Cell Mol Med,* 14(3), 600-607.

32. Dufault, R., & Gilbert, S.G. (2011). Implications of organophosphate (OP) pesticides in food grain. *Poster Presented at Society of Toxicology Conference: 6-10 March 2011; Washington D.C.* Retrieved from www.foodingredient.info/images/SOT_Poster_for_2011_Conference.pdf

33. Pasca, S.P., Nemes, B., Vlase, L., Gagyi, C.E., Dronca, E., Miu, A.C., & Dronca, M. (2006). High levels of homocysteine and low serum paraoxanase 1 arlesterase activity in children with autism. *Life Sci,* 78, 2244-2248.

34. Bacchetti, T., Vignini, A., Giulietti, A., et al. (2015). Higher levels of oxidized low density lipoproteins in Alzheimer's disease patients: roles for platelet activating factor acetyl hydrolase and paraoxonase-1. *Journal of Alzheimer's Disease,* 46(1):179-186.

35. Cervellati, C., Trentini, A., Romani, A., et al. (2015). Serum paraoxonase and arylesterase activities of paraoxonase-1 (PON-1), mild cognitive impairment, and 2-year conversion to dementia: a pilot study. *Journal of Neurochemistry,* 135(2):395-401.

36. Zaganas, I., Kapetanaki, S., Mastorodemos, V., et al. (2013). Linking pesticide exposure and dementia: what is the evidence? *Toxicology,* 307:3-11.

37. Hernandez, A.F., Gonzalez-Alzaga, B., Lopez-Flores, I., & Lacasana, M. (2016). Systemic reviews on neurodevelopmental and neurodegenerative disorders linked to pesticide exposure: methodological features and impact on risk assessment. *Environment International,* 92-93:657-679.

38. Costa, L.G., Vitalone, A., Cole, T.B., & Furlong, C. E. (2005). Modulation of paraoxonase (PON1) activity. *Biochem Pharmacol,* 69, 541-550. Retrieved from http://perweb.firat.edu.tr/personel/yayinlar/fua_870/870_21956.pdf

39. Huen, K., Harley, K., & Brooks, J. et al. (2009). Developmental changes in PON1 enzyme activity in young children and effects of PON1 polymorphisms. *Environmental Health Perspectives,* 117(10):1632-1638. Retrieved from www.ncbi.nlm.nih.gov/ pmc/articles/PMC2790521/pdf/ehp-117-1632.pdf

40. Shelton, J.F., Geraghty, E.M., Tancredi, D.J., Delwiche, L.D., Schmidt, R.J., Ritz, B., Hansen, R.L., & Hertz-Picciotto, I. Neurodevelopmental disorders and prenatal residential proximity to agricultural pesticides: the CHARGE study. *Environmental Health Perspectives,* epub. Retrieved from http://ehp.niehs.nih.gov/wp-content/uploads/advpub/2014/6/ehp.1307044.pdf

41. Fitzpatrick, A.L., Kuller, L.H., Ives, D.G., et al. (2004). Incidence and prevalence of dementia in the Cardiovascular Health Study. *Journal of the American Geriatrics Society,* 52(2):195-204.

42. Cakatay, U., Kayali, R., & Uzun, H. (2008). Relation of plasma protein oxidation parameters and paraoxonase activity in the ageing population. *Clinical and Experimental Medicine,* 8(1):51-57.

43. Seres, I., Paragh, G., Deschene, E., Fulop, T., & Khalil, A. (2004). Study of factors influencing the decreased HDL associated PON1 activity with aging. *Experimental Gerontology,* 39(1):59-66.

44. United States Department of Agriculture. (2014). *National nutrient database.* Retrieved from www.ars.usda.gov/Services/docs.htm?docid=8964

45. Mahaffey, K.R., Gartside, P.S., & Glueck, C.J. (1986). Blood lead levels and dietary calcium intake in 1 to 11 year-old children: the second national health and nutrition examination survey, 1976 to 1980. *Pediatrics ,* 78, 257–262.

46. Shannon, M., & Graef, J.W. (1996). Lead intoxication in children with pervasive developmental disorders. *J Toxicol Clin Toxicol,* 34, 177-181.

47. Eubig, P.A., Aguiar, A., & Schantz, S.L. (2010). Lead and PCBs as risk factors for attention deficit/hyperactivity disorder. *Environ Health Perspect,* 118, 1654-1667. Retrieved from www.ncbi.nlm.nih.gov/pmc/articles/PMC3002184/

48. Chin-Chan, M., Navarro-Yepes, J., Quintanilla-Vega, B. (2015). Environmental pollutants as risk factors for neurodegenerative disorders: Alzheimer and Parkinson diseases. *Frontiers in Cellular Neuroscience,* 9:124. Retrieved from www.ncbi.nlm.nih.gov/ pmc/articles/PMC4392704/pdf/fncel-09-00124.pdf

49. Coyle, P., Philcox, J.C., Carey, L.C., & Rofe, A.M. (2002). Metallothionein: the multipurpose protein. *Cell Mol Life Sci,* 59, 627–647.

50. Dufault, R., Schnoll, R., Lukiw, W.J., LeBlanc, B., Cornett, C., Patrick, L., Wallinga, D., Gilbert, S.G., & Crider, R. (2009). Mercury exposure, nutritional deficiencies and metabolic disruptions may affect learning in children. *Behavioral and Brain Functions,* 5:44. Retrieved from www.ncbi.nlm.nih.gov/pmc/articles/PMC2773803/#!po=76.0417

51. Faber, S., Zinn, G.M., Kern, J.C., & Kingston, H.M. (2009). The plasma zinc/serum copper ratio as a biomarker in children with autism spectrum disorders. *Biomarkers,* 14, 171–180.

52. Blaylock, R.L. (2009). A possible central mechanism in autism spectrum disorders, part 2: immunoexcitotoxicity. *Altern Ther Health Med,* 5, 60–67.

53. Bjorklund, G. (2013). The role of zinc and copper in autism spectrum disorders. *Acta Neurobiol Exp (Wars).* 73(2), 225-236.

54. Yu, W.H., Lukiw, W.J., Bergeron, C., Niznik, H.B., & Fraser, P.E. (2001). Metallothionein III is reduced in Alzheimer's disease. *Brain Research,* 894(1):37-45.

55. Pal, A., Kumar, A., Prasad, R. (2014). Predictive association of copper metabolism proteins in Alzheimer's disease and Parkinson's disease: a preliminary perspective. *Biometals,* 27(1):25-31.

56. Ventriglia, M., Brewer, G.J., Simonelli, I., et al. (2015). Zinc in Alzheimer's disease: a meta-analysis of serum, plasma, and cerebral spinal fluid status. *Journal of Alzheimer's Disease,* 46(1):75-87.

57. Ward, N.I., Soulsbury, K., Zettel, V.H., Colquhoun, I.D., Bunday, S., & Barnes, B. (1990).

The influence of the chemical additive tartrazine on the zinc status of hyperactive children-a double-blind placebo-controlled study. *J Nutr Med,* 1, 51–57.

58. Ward, N.I. (1997). Assessment of chemical factors in relation to child hyperactivity. *J Nutr Environ Med.* 7, 333–342. Retrieved from www.feingold.org/Research/PDFstudies/Ward97.pdf

59. Yasuda, H., & Tsutsui, T. (2013). Assessment of infantile mineral imbalances in autism spectrum disorders (ASDs). *Int J Environ Res Pub Health,* 10(11), 6027-6043. Retrieved from www.ncbi.nlm.nih.gov/pmc/articles/PMC3863885/

60. Federman, D.G., Kirsner, R.S., Federman, G.S. (1997). Pica: are you hungry for the facts? *Conn Med,* 61(4), 207-209.

61. Chatzimavroudis, G., Christopoulos, P., Atmatzidis, S., Papadakis, G., Nalbanti, P., Papaaziogas, B., Koutelidakis, I., Atmatzidis, K. (2011). Pica: an uncommon cause of acute abdominal pain in children. *Indian J Pediatr,* 78(7), 886-887.

62. Vega-Franco, L., Hernandez-Romo, A., Meza Camiacho, C., Calderon, F. (1976). [Concentration of lead in the blood of children with hyperkinesis]. *Bol Med Hosp Infant Mex,* 33(5), 1143-1149.

63. Baloh, R., Sturm, R., Green, B., Gleser, G. (1975). Neuropsychological effects of chronic asymptomatic increased lead absorption: a controlled study. *Arch Neurol,* 32(5), 326-330.

64. Clark, B., Vandermeer, B., Simonetti, A., Buka, I. (2010). Is lead a concern in Canadian autistic children? *Paediatr Child Health,* 15(1), 17-22. Retrieved from www.ncbi.nlm.nih.gov/pmc/articles/PMC2827318/pdf/pch15017.pdf

65. Dufault, R. (2014, April). Dufault, R. (2014, April). The medicine of food. In J. Barreiro (Chair), *Patterns of health and wellbeing.* Symposium conducted at the Smithsonian Institute National Museum of the American Indian. Retrieved from https://www.youtube.com/watch?v=IwapwKitM0k

66. Feero, W.G., & Gutmacher, A.E. (2014). Genomics, personalized medicine, and pediatrics. *Academic Pediatrics,* 14(1):14-22. Retrieved from www.ncbi.nlm.nih.gov/ pmc/articles/PMC4227880/pdf/nihms-504130.pdf

67. Torano, E.G., Garcia, M.G., Fernandez-Morera, J.L., Nino-Garcia, P., & Fernandez, A.F. (2016). The impact of external factors on the epigenome: *in utero* and over lifetime. *Biomed Research International,* 2016: 2568635. Retrieved from www.ncbi.nlm.nih.gov/ pmc/articles/PMC4887632/pdf/BMRI2016-2568635.pdf

68. Bjorling-Poulsen, M., Andersen, H.R., & Grandjean, P. (2008). Potential developmental neurotoxicity of pesticides used in Europe. *Environmental Health,* 7:50. Retrieved from www.ehjournal.net/content/7/1/50

69. Bouchard, M.F., Bellinger, D.C., & Wright, R.O. (2010). Attention-deficit hyperactivity disorder and urinary metabolites of organophosphate pesticides. *Pediatrics,* 125:e1270-e1277. Retrieved from http://pediatrics.aappublications.org/content/125/6/e1270.full

70. Harari, R., Julvez, J., Murata, K., Barr, D., Bellinger, D., Debes, F., & Grandjean, P. (2010). Neurobehavioral deficits and increased blood pressure in school-age children prenatally exposed to pesticides. *Environmental Health Perspectives,* 118, 890-6. Retrieved from www.ncbi.nlm.nih.gov/pmc/articles/PMC2898869/pdf/ehp-118-890.pdf

71. Jurewicz, J., & Hanke, W. (2008). Prenatal and childhood exposure to pesticides and

neurobehavioral development: review of epidemiological studies. *International Journal of Occupational Medicine and Environmental Health,* 21, 121-32. Retrieved from www .degruyter.com/view/j/ijmh.2008.21.issue-2/v10001-008-0014-z/v10001-008-0014-z.xml

72. Bouchard, M.F., Chevrier, J., Harley, K.G., Kogut, K., Vedar, M., Calderon, N., Trujillo, C., Johnson, C., Bradman, A., Barr, D., & Eskenazi, B. (2011). Prenatal exposure to organophosphate pesticides and IQ in 7-year-old children. *Environmental Health Perspectives,* 119, 1189-95. Retrieved from www.ncbi.nlm.nih.gov/pmc/articles/PMC3237357/pdf/ehp.1003185.pdf

73. Perera, F.P., Rauh, V., Whyatt, R.M., Tang, D., Tsai, W.Y., Bernert, J.T., Tu, Y.H., Andrews, H., Barr, D.B., Camann, D.E., Diaz, D., Dietrich, J., Reyes, A. & Kinney, P.L. (2005). A summary of recent findings on birth outcomes and developmental effects of prenatal ETS, PAH, and pesticide exposures. *Neurotoxicology,* 26, 573-587.

74. Nevison, C.D. (2014). A comparison of temporal trends in United States autism prevalence trends in suspected environmental factors. *Environmental Health,* 13, 1, Retrieved from www.ehjournal.net/content/13/1/73/abstract

CHAPTER 3

1. Environmental Protection Agency. (2016). *Why we use pesticides.* www.epa.gov/safepest-control/why-we-use-pesticides

2. Environmental Protection Agency. (2015). *Chlorine bleach.* Retrieved from www.epa.gov/kidshometour/products/bleach.htm

3. Environmental Protection Agency. (2006). *Reregistration eligibility decision (RED) for chlorine dioxide and sodium chlorite (case 4023).* Retrieved from www.epa.gov/pesticides/reregistration/REDs/chlorine_dioxide_red.pdf

4. United States Department of Agriculture. (2011). *Guidance: the use of chlorine materials in organic production and handling.* Retrieved from www.ams.usda.gov/AMSv1.0/getfile?dDocName=STELPRDC5090760

5. Institute of Food Technologists. (2006). *Antimicrobial resistance: implications for the food system.* Retrieved from www.fws.gov/fisheries/aadap/PDF/IFT%20-%20InPress%20-%20Antimicrobial-Expert-Report%20june%2006.pdf

6. Murray, G.E., Tobin, R.S., Junkins, B., Kushner, D.J. (1984). Effect of chlorination on antibiotic resistance profiles of sewage-related bacteria. *Appl Environ Microbial,* 48(1), 73-77. Retrieved from www.ncbi.nlm.nih.gov/pmc/articles/PMC240314/pdf/aem00152-0081.pdf

7. Yuan, Q-B., Guo, M-T., Yang, J. (2015). Fate of antibiotic resistant bacteria and genes during wastewater chlorination: implication for antibiotic resistance control. *PLoS ONE,* 10(3), e0119403. Retrieved from www.plosone.org/article/fetchObject.action?uri=info:doi/10.1371/journal.pone.0119403&representation=PDF

8. United States Center for Disease Control and Prevention. (2016). *Antibiotic/antimicrobial resistance: biggest threats.* www.cdc.gov/drugresistance/biggest_threats.html

9. Montana Department of Agriculture. (2004). *Pest management for grain storage and fumigation.* Retrieved from www.pesticides.montana.edu/Reference/FumSeed.pdf

10. Food and Agriculture Organization (FAO). (2006). Chlorine *monograph.* Retrieved from www.fao.org/ag/agn/jecfa-additives/specs/Monograph1/Additive-126.pdf

11. International Program on Chemical Safety (INCHEM). *Chlorine.* Retrieved from 9ttp://www.inchem.org/documents/jecfa/jecmono/v20je09.htm

12. United States Department of Agriculture. (2006). *Pesticide data program annual summary calendar year 2004.* Retrieved from www.ams.usda.gov/sites/default/files/media/2004%20PDP%20Annual%20Summary.pdf

13. United States Department of Agriculture. (2007). *Pesticide data program annual summary calendar year 2006.* Retrieved from www.ams.usda.gov/sites/default/files/media/2006%20PDP%20Annual%20Summary.pdf

14. United States Department of Agriculture. (2006). *Pesticide data program annual summary calendar year 2005.* Retrieved from www.ams.usda.gov/sites/default/files/media/2005%20PDP%20Annual%20Summary.pdf

15. United States Department of Agriculture. (2008). *Pesticide data program annual summary calendar year 2007.* Retrieved from www.ams.usda.gov/sites/default/files/media/2007%20PDP%20Annual%20Summary.pdf

16. United States Department of Agriculture. (2009). *Pesticide data program annual summary calendar year 2008.* Retrieved from www.ams.usda.gov/sites/default/files/media/2008%20PDP%20Annual%20Summary.pdf

17. Dufault, R., & Gilbert, S.G. (2011). *Implications of organophosphate (OP) pesticides in food grain.* Poster presented at the meeting of the Society of Toxicology, Washington, D.C. Available at www.foodingredient.info/images/SOT_Poster_for_2011_Conference.pdf

18. United States Department of Agriculture. (2014). *Pesticide data program annual summary calendar year 2012.* Retrieved from www.ams.usda.gov/sites/default/files/media/2012%20PDP%20Annual%20Summary.pdf

19. United States Department of Agriculture. (2011). *Pesticide data program annual summary calendar year 2009.* Retrieved from www.ams.usda.gov/sites/default/files/media/2009%20PDP%20Annual%20Summary.pdf

20. United States Department of Agriculture. (2012). *Pesticide data program annual summary calendar year 2010.* Retrieved from www.ams.usda.gov/sites/default/files/media/2010%20PDP%20Annual%20Summary.pdf

21. United States Department of Agriculture. (2016). *Pesticide data program.* www.ams.usda.gov/datasets/pdp

22. Rehm, C.D., Penalvo, J.L., Afshin, A., & Mozaffarian, D. (2016). Dietary intake among U.S. adults, 1999-2012. *JAMA,* 315(23):2542-2553. file:///C:/Users/rdufault/Downloads/JOI160065supp1_prod%20(1).pdf

23. United States Department of Agriculture. (2015). *Food availability per capita data system.* Retrieved from www.ers.usda.gov/data-products/food-availability-%28per-capita%29-data-system.aspx#.Ud3WT3-kBTY

24. Dufault, R., Lukiw, W.J., Crider, R., Schnoll, R., Wallinga, D., & Deth, R. (2012). A macroepigenetic approach to identify the factors responsible for the autism epidemic in the United States. *Clinical Epigenetics,* 4:6. Retrieved from www.clinicalepigeneticsjournal.com/content/4/1/6

25. United States Department of Agriculture. (2016). *PDP databases and annual summaries.* Retrieved from www.ams.usda.gov/datasets/pdp/pdpdata

26. United States Department of Agriculture. (2016). *Pesticide data program annual summary calendar year 2014.* Retrieved from www.ams.usda.gov/sites/default/files/media/2014%20PDP%20Annual%20Summary.pdf

27. Balinova, A., Mladenova, R., Obretenchev, D. (2006). Effect of grain storage and processing on chlorpyrifos-methyl and pirimiphos-methyl residues on post-harvest treated wheat with regard to baby food safety requirements. *Food Addit Contam,* 23(4), 391-397.

28. Skerritt, J.H., Guihot, S.L., Hill, A.S., Desmarchelier, J., Gore, P.J. (1996). Analysis of organophosphate, pyrethroid, and methoprene residues in wheat end products and milling fractions by immunoassay. *Analytical Techniques and Instrumentation.* 73(5), 605-612. Retrieved from www.aaccnet.org/publications/cc/backissues/1996/Documents/73_605.pdf

29. United States Public Health Service, Agency for Toxic Substances and Disease Registry. (2006). Interaction profile for: chlorpyrifos, lead, mercury, and methylmercury. Retrieved from www.atsdr.cdc.gov/interactionprofiles/IP-11/ip11.pdf

30. Lentz, T.J., Dotson, G.S., Williams, P.R.D., et al. (2015). Aggregate exposure and cumulative risk assessment—integrating occupational and non-occupational health risk factors. *Journal of Occupational and Environmental Hygiene,* 12:S112-S126. Retrieved from www.ncbi.nlm.nih.gov/pmc/articles/PMC4654690/pdf/uoeh-12-S112.pdf

31. Wason, S.C., Smith, T.J., Perry, M.J., & Levy, J.I. (2012). Using physiologically-based pharmacokinetic models to incorporate chemical and non-chemical stressors into cumulative risk assessment: a case study of pesticide exposures. *International Journal of Environmental Research and Public Health,* 9: 1971-1983. Retrieved from www.ncbi.nlm.nih.gov/pmc/articles/PMC3386599/pdf/ijerph-09-01971.pdf

32. Ray, P.D., Yosim, A., Fry, R. C. (2014). Incorporating epigenetic data into the risk assessment process for toxic metals arsenic, cadmium, chromium, lead, and mercury: strategies and challenges. *Front Genet,* 5:201 Retrieved from www.ncbi.nlm.nih.gov/pmc/articles/PMC4100550/pdf/fgene-05-00201.pdf

33. Hirtz, D., Thurman, D.J., Gwinn-Hardy, K., Mohamed, M., Chaudhuri, A.R., & Zalutsky, R. (2007). How common are the "common" neurologic disorders? *Neurology,* 68(5):326-337. Retrieved from http://citeseerx.ist.psu.edu/viewdoc/download?doi=10.1.1.452.7479&rep=rep1&type=pdf

34. Centers for Disease Control and Prevention. (2016). *Alzheimer's disease.* Retrieved from www.cdc.gov/aging/aginginfo/alzheimers.htm

35. Hurd, M.D., Martorell, P., Delavande, A., Mullen, K.J., & Langa, K.M. (2013). Monetary costs of dementia in the United States. *New England Journal of Medicine,* 368(14):1326-1334. Retrieved from www.ncbi.nlm.nih.gov/pmc/articles/PMC3959992/pdf/nihms464155.pdf

36. Mayeux, R., & Stern, Y. (2012). Epidemiology of Alzheimer's disease. *Cold Spring Harbor Perspectives in Medicine,* 2(8): a006239. Retrieved from www.ncbi.nlm.nih.gov/pmc/articles/PMC3405821/pdf/cshperspectmed-ALZ-a006239.pdf

37. Hayden, K.M., Norton, M.C., Darcey, D., et al. Occupational exposure to pesticides

increases the risk of incident AD: the Cache County Study. Neurology, 74:1524-1530. Retrieved from www.ncbi.nlm.nih.gov/pmc/articles/PMC2875926/pdf/7635.pdf

38. Liu, C-C., Kanekiyo, T., Xu, H., & Bu, G. (2013). Apolipoprotein E and Alzheimer disease: risk, mechanisms, and therapy. *Nature Reviews Neurology*, 9(2):106-118. Retrieved from www.ncbi.nlm.nih.gov/pmc/articles/PMC3726719/pdf/nihms492068.pdf

39. Downer, B., Zanjani, F., & Fardo, D.W. (20114). The relationship between midlife and late life alcohol consumption, APOE e4 and the decline in learning and memory among older adults. Alcohol and Alcoholism, 49(1):17-22. Retrieved from www.ncbi.nlm.nih .gov/pmc/articles/PMC3865814/pdf/agt144.pdf

40. Yegambaram, M., Manivannan, B., Beach, T.G., & Halden, R.U. (2015). Role of environmental contaminants in the etiology of Alzheimer's disease: a review. *Current Alzheimer Research*, 12, 116-146. Retrieved from www.ncbi.nlm.nih.gov/pmc/articles/ PMC4428475/pdf/CAR-12-116.pdf

41. Chin-Chan, M., Navarro-Yepes, J., & Quintanilla-Vega, B. (2015). Environmental pollutants as risk factors for neurodegenerative disorders: Alzheimer and Parkinson diseases. *Frontiers in Cellular Neuroscience*, 9:123. Retrieved from www.ncbi.nlm.nih.gov/pmc/articles/PMC4392704/pdf/fncel-09-00124.pdf

42. National Institutes of Health. (2016). *Focus on Parkinson's disease research.* www.ninds .nih.gov/research/parkinsonsweb/index.htm

43. Narayan, S., Liew, Z., Paul, K., et al. (2013). Household organophosphate pesticide use and Parkinson's disease. *International Journal of Epidemiology*, 42:1476-1485. Retrieved from www.ncbi.nlm.nih.gov/pmc/articles/PMC3807617/pdf/dyt170.pdf

44. United States National Library of Medicine. (2016). *Metabolic disorders.* www.nlm .nih.gov/medlineplus/metabolicdisorders.html

45. Seyfried, T.N., Flores, R.E., Poff, A.M., & Agostino, D.P.D. (2014). Cancer as a metabolic disease: implications for novel therapeutics. *Carcinogenesis*, 35(3):515-527. Retrieved from www.ncbi.nlm.nih.gov/pmc/articles/PMC3941741/pdf/bgt480.pdf

46. Coller, H.A. (2014). Is cancer a metabolic disease? *American Journal of Pathology*, 184(1):4-17. Retrieved from http://ajp.amjpathol.org/article/S0002-9440(13)00653-6/pdf

47. Heron, M. (2016). Deaths: leading causes for 2013. *National Vital Statistics Reports*, 65(2):1-95. Retrieved from www.cdc.gov/nchs/data/nvsr/nvsr65/nvsr65_02.pdf

48. National Institute of Health. (2013). *Diabetes, heart disease and stroke.* Retrieved from www.niddk.nih.gov/health-information/health-topics/Diabetes/diabetes-heart-disease-stroke/Pages/index.aspx

49. Eranti, A., Kerola, T., Aro, A.L., et al. (2016). Diabetes, glucose tolerance, and the risk of sudden cardiac death. *BMC Cardiovascular Disease*, 16:51. Retrieved from www.ncbi.nlm.nih.gov/pmc/articles/PMC4765126/pdf/12872_2016_Article_231.pdf

50. Lukaszewicz-Hussain, A. (2013). [Serum glucose concentration in subacute intoxication with chlorpyrifos organophosphate insecticides]. *Medycyna Pracy*, 64(4):527-531.

51. Lasram, M.M., El-Golli, N., Lamine, A.J., et al. (2015). Changes in glucose metabolism and reversion of genes expression in the liver of insulin-resistant rats exposed to malathion. The protective effects of N-acetylcysteine. *General and Comparative Endocrinology*, 215:88-97.

52. Raafat, N., Abass, M.A., & Salem, H.M. (2012). Malathion exposure and insulin resistance among a group of farmers in Al-Sharkia governorate. *Clinical Biochemistry,* 45(18):1591-1595.

53. Centers for Disease Control and Prevention. (2016). *NHANES.* Retrieved from www.cdc.gov/nchs/nhanes/

CHAPTER 4

1. Dufault, R., LeBlanc, B., Schnoll, R., Cornett, C., Schweitzer, L., Wallinga, D., Hightower, J., Patrick, L., & Lukiw, W.J. (2009). Mercury from chlor-alkali plants: measured concentrations in food product sugar. *Environmental Health,* 8:2. Retrieved from www.ehjournal .net/content/8/1/2

2. Dufault, R., Schnoll, R., Lukiw, W.J., LeBlanc, B., Cornett, C., Patrick, L., Wallinga, D., Gilbert, S.G., & Crider, R. (2009). Mercury exposure, nutritional deficiencies and metabolic disruptions may affect learning in children. *Behavioral and Brain Functions,* 5:44. Retrieved from www.ncbi.nlm.nih.gov/pmc/articles/PMC2773803/#!po=76.0417

3. Islam, M.S., Ahmed, M.K., & Habibullah-Al-Mamun, M. (2014). Heavy metals in cereals and pulses: health implications in Bangladesh. *J Agric Food Chem,*

4. Hsu, W.H., Jiang, S.J., & Sahayam, A.C. (2013). Determination of Cu, As, Hg, and Pb in vegetable oils by electrothermal vaporization inductively coupled plasma mass spectrometry with palladium nanoparticles as modifier. *Talanta,* 117, 268-272.

5. Kahn, K., Khan, H., Lu, Y., Ihsanullah, I., Nawab, J., Khan, S., Shah, N.S., Shamshad, I., & Maryam, A. (2014). Evaluation of toxicological risk of foodstuffs contaminated with heavy metals in Swat, Pakistan. *Ecotoxicol Environ Saf,* 108, 224-232.

6. Eom, S.Y., Choi, S.H., Ahn, S.J., Kim, D.K., Kim, D.W., Lim, J.A., Choi, B.S., Shin, H.J., Yun, S.W., Yoon, H.J., Kim, Y.M., Hong, Y.S., Yun, Y.W., Sohn, S.J., Kim, H., Park, K.S., Pyo, H.S., Kim, H., Oh, S.Y., Kim, J., Lee, S.A., Ha, M., Kwon, H.J., & Park, J.D. (2014). Reference levels of blood mercury and association with metabolic syndrome in Korean adults. *Int Arch Occup Environ Health,* 87(5), 501-513.

7. Ettinger, A.S., Bovet, P., Plange-Rhule, J., Forrester, T.E., Lambert, E.V., Lupoli, N., Shine, J., Dugas, L.R., Shoham, D., Durazo-Arvizu, R.A., Cooper, R.S., & Luke, A. (2014). Distribution of metals exposure and associations with cardiometabolic risk factors in the "Modeling the Epidemiologic Transition Study." *Eviron Health,* 13:90. Retrieved from www.ehjournal.net/content/pdf/1476-069X-13-90.pdf

8. Poursafa, P., Ataee, E., Motlagh, M.E., Ardalan, G., Tajadini, M.H., Yazdi, M., & Kelishadi, R. (2014). Association of serum lead and mercury level with cardiometabolic risk factors and liver enzymes in a nationally representative sample of adolescents: the CASPIAN-III study. *Environ Sci Pollut Res Int,* 21(23), 13496-13502.

9. European Feed Ingredients Safety Certification. (2013). *Sector reference document on the manufacturing of safe feed materials from oilseed crushing and vegetable oil refining.* www.efisc.eu/data/1377527038FEDIOL percent20- percent20version percent203.0 percent20- percent20Sector percent20ref percent20doc percent20on percent20oilseed percent20crushing percent20and percent20veg percent20oil percent20refining percent20version percent203.0.pdf

10. Abd El-Salam, A.S.M., Doheim, M.A., Sitohy, M.Z., & Ramadan, M.F. (2011). Deacidifi-

cation of high-acid olive oil. *J Food Processing & Technology*, S5-001. Retrieved from http://omicsonline.org/deacidification-of-high-acid-olive-oil-2157-7110.S5-001.pdf

11. Canola Council. (2014). *Canola seed and oil processing.* Retrieved from www.canolacouncil.org/media/515283/canola_seed_and_oil_processing.pdf

12. Simopoulos, A.P.(2008). The omega-6/omega-3 fatty acid ratio, genetic variation, and cardiovascular disease. *Asia Pac J Clin Nutr,* 17 (Suppl 1), 131-134. Retrieved from http://apjcn.nhri.org.tw/server/apjcn/17/s1/131.pdf

13. United States Department of Agriculture. (2014). *Food availability (per capita) data system.* Retrieved from www.ers.usda.gov/data-products/food-availability-per-capita-data-system/

14. Zeldenrust, R.S. (2012). *Edible oil processing: alkali refining.* Retrieved from http://lipidlibrary.aocs.org/processing/alkrefining/index.htm

15. El-Salam, A.S., Doheim, M.A., Sitohy, M.Z., & Ramadan, M.F. (2011). Deacidification of high-acid olive oil. *Food Processing & Technology,* S5, 1-7. Retrieved from http://omicsonline.org/deacidification-of-high-acid-olive-oil-2157-7110.S5-001.pdf

16. Mounts, T.L. (1981). Chemical and physical effects of processing fats and oils. *Journal of the American Oil Chemists' Society,* 58(1), 51-54A. Retrieved from http://naldc.nal.usda.gov/naldc/download.xhtml?id=26334&content=PDF

17. Dufault, R., Lukiw, W.J., Crider, R., Schnoll, R., Wallinga, D., & Deth, R. (2012). A macroepigenetic approach to identify the factors responsible for the autism epidemic in the United States. *Clinical Epigenetics,* 4:6. Retrieved from www.clinicalepigeneticsjournal.com/content/4/1/6

18. Dufault, R. (2014, April). Dufault, R. (2014, April). The medicine of food. In J. Barreiro (Chair), *Patterns of health and wellbeing.* Symposium conducted at the Smithsonian Institute National Museum of the American Indian. Retrieved from www.youtube.com/watch?v=IwapwKitM0k

19. Butzen, S., & Hobbs, T. (2002). Corn processing III: wet milling. *Crop Insights,* 12(15), 1-6.

20. Guzman-Maldonado, H., & Paredes-Lopez, O. (1995). Amylolytic enzymes and products derived from starch: a review. *Critical Reviews in Food Science and Nutrition,* 35(5), 373-403.

21. Lurgi Life Science GmbH. High Fructose Syrup Production-Process and Economics. In *Proceedings of International Conference on Value-Added Products for the Sugar Industry.* Baton Rouge; 1999.

22. Institute of Medicine. (2003). *Food Chemicals Codex* 5th edition. Washington DC: National Academies Press; 2003.

23. World Health Organization.(2005). *Evaluation of certain food additives.* Retrieved from http://whqlibdoc.who.int/trs/WHO_TRS_928.pdf

24. Rideout, K. (2010). Comment on the paper by Dufault et al.: Mercury in foods containing high fructose corn syrup in Canada. *Environmental Health,* 8:2. Retrieved from www.ehjournal.net/content/8/1/2/comments#418684

25. Wallinga, D., Sorensen, J., Mottl, P., & Yablon, B. (2009). *Not so sweet: missing mercury and high fructose corn syrup.* Retrieved from www.iatp.org/files/421_2_105026.pdf

26. Dufault, R., Berg, Z., Crider, R., Schnoll R., Wetsit, L., Two Bulls, W., Gilbert, S., Kingston, S., Wolle, M., Rahman, M., & Laks, D. (2015). Blood inorganic mercury is directly associated with glucose levels in the human population and may be linked to processed food intake. *Integrative Molecular Medicine,* 2(3), 166-179. Retrieved from http://oatext.com/pdf/IMM-2-134.pdf

27. Cordain L., Eaton S.B., Sebastian A., Mann N., Lindeberg S., Watkins B.A., O'Keefe J.H., & Brand-Miller J. (2005). Origins and evolution of the western diet: health implications for the 21st century. *Am. J. Clin. Nutr,* 81, 341–354. Retrieved from http://ajcn.nutrition.org/content/81/2/341.full.pdf

28. United States Code of Federal Regulations. (2014). *Part 74: listing of color additives subject to certification.* Retrieved from www.ecfr.gov/cgi-bin/retrieveECFR?gp=&SID=56f57bc56bb3686c1cc9c387d675d1d3&n=pt21.1.74&r=PART&ty=HTML#se21.1.74_1101]

29. United Kingdom Food Standards Agency. (2011). *FSA advice to parents on food colors and hyperactivity.* Retrieved from http://tna.europarchive.org/20120209132957/www.food.gov.uk/safereating/chemsafe/additivesbranch/colours/hyper/

30. Curran, L. (2010, July 21). EU places warning labels on foods containing dyes. *Food Safety News.* Retrieved from www.foodsafetynews.com/2010/07/eu-places-warning-labels-on-foods-containing-dyes/#.V3ItjfkrKM8

31. Ward, N. (1997). Assessment of chemical factors in relation to child hyperactivity. *J Nutr Environ Med,* 7:333-342.

32. Ward, N.I., Soulsbury, K.A., Zettel, V.H., Colquhoun, I.D., Bunday, S., & Barnes, B. (1990). The influence of the chemical additive tartrazine on the zinc status of hyperactive children-a double-blind placebo controlled study. *J Nutr Med* 1990, 1(1), 51-57.

33. Bateman, B., Warner, J.O., Hutchinson, E., Dean, T., Rowlandson, P., Gant, C., Grundy, J., Fitzgerald, C., & Stevenson, J. (2004). The effects of a double blind, placebo controlled artificial food colorings and sodium benzoate preservative challenge on hyperactivity in a general population sample of preschool children. *Arch Dis Child,* 89, 506-511. Retrieved from www.ncbi.nlm.nih.gov/pmc/articles/PMC1719942/pdf/v089p00506.pdf

34. McCann Food additives and hyperactive behavior in 3-year-old and 8/9-year-old children in the community: a randomized, double-blinded placebo-controlled trial. *Lancet* 2007, 370(9598), 1560-1567. www.feingold.org/Research/PDFstudies/Stevenson2007.pdf

35. Thirumoorthy, N., Sunder, A.S., Kumar, K.T.M., Kumar, M.S., Ganesh, G.N.K., & Chatterjee, M. (2011). A review of metallothionein isoforms and their role in pathophysiology. *World Journal of Surgical Oncology,* 9:54. Retrieved from www.wjso.com/content/pdf/1477-7819-9-54.pdf

36. United States Food and Drug Administration. (2003). *Color additives: FDA's regulatory process and historical perspectives.* Retrieved from www.fda.gov/ForIndustry/ColorAdditives/RegulatoryProcessHistoricalPerspectives/

37. Griffiths, J.C. (2005). Coloring foods & beverages. *Food Technology,* 59(6), 38-44. Retrieved from www.ift.org/~/media/Food percent20Technology/pdf/2005/05/0505feat_coloringfoods.pdf

38. United States Code of Federal Regulations. (2014). *Part 73: listing of color additives exempt from certification.* Retrieved from www.accessdata.fda.gov/scripts/cdrh/cfdocs/cfCFR/CFRSearch.cfm?CFRPart=73&showFR=1

39. Koru, E. (2012). Earth food spirulina (arthrospira): production and quality standards. In Prof. Yehia El-Samragy (ed.), *Food Additive* (pp. 191-202). Retrieved from http://cdn.intechopen.com/pdfs-wm/28916.pdf

40. Al-Dhabi, N.A. (2013). Heavy metal analysis in commercial *Spirulina* products for human consumption. Saudi *Journal of Biological Sciences*, 20, 383-388. Retrieved from www.sciencedirect.com/science/article/pii/S1319562X13000430

41. Food and Agriculture Organization. (2004). *Compendium of Food Additive Specifications, Addendum 12.* Retrieved from ftp://ftp.fao.org/docrep/fao/007/y5777e/y5777e00.pdf

42. United States Food and Drug Administration. (2014). *Overview of food ingredients, additives and colors.* www.fda.gov/Food/IngredientsPackagingLabeling/FoodAdditivesIngredients/ucm094211.htm

43. Mahaffey, K.R., Gartside, P.S., & Glueck, C.J. (1986). Blood lead levels and dietary calcium intake in 1 to 11 year-old children: the second national health and nutrition examination survey, 1976 to 1980. *Pediatrics* , 78, 257-262.

44. Shannon, M., & Graef, J.W. (1996). Lead intoxication in children with pervasive developmental disorders. *J Toxicol Clin Toxicol*, 34, 177-181.

45. Eubig, P.A., Aguiar, A., & Schantz, S.L. (2010). Lead and PCBs as risk factors for attention deficit/hyperactivity disorder. *Environ Health Perspect*, 118, 1654-1667. Retrieved from www.ncbi.nlm.nih.gov/pmc/articles/PMC3002184/

46. Chin-Chan, M., Navarro-Yepes, J., Quintanilla-Vega, B. (2015). Environmental pollutants as risk factors for neurodegenerative disorders: Alzheimer and Parkinson diseases. *Frontiers in Cellular Neuroscience*, 9:124. Retrieved from www.ncbi.nlm.nih.gov/pmc/articles/PMC4392704/pdf/fncel-09-00124.pdf

47. Food and Agriculture Organization. (2007). *Carrageenan monograph.* Retrieved from www.fao.org/ag/agn/jecfa-additives/specs/monograph4/additive-117-m4.pdf

48. Food and Agriculture Organization. (2006). *Citric acid monograph.* Retrieved from www.fao.org/ag/agn/jecfa-additives/specs/Monograph1/Additive-135.pdf

49. Food and Agriculture Organization. (2006). *Monosodium glutamate monograph.* Retrieved from www.fao.org/ag/agn/jecfa-additives/specs/Monograph1/Additive-292.pdf

50. United States Code of Federal Regulations. (2014). *Sodium benzoate.* Retrieved from www.accessdata.fda.gov/scripts/cdrh/cfdocs/cfcfr/CFRSearch.cfm?fr=184.1733

51. Joint FAO/WHO Expert Committee on Food Additives. (2002). *Limit test for heavy metals in food additive specifications: explanatory note.* Retrieved from www.fao.org/fileadmin/templates/agns/pdf/jecfa/2002-09-10_Explanatory_note_Heavy_Metals.pdf

52. Food and Agricultural Organization of the United Nations. (2004). *Compendium of food additive specifications.* Retrieved from ftp://ftp.fao.org/es/esn/jecfa/addendum_12.pdf

53. Food and Agricultural Organization of the United Nations. (2006). *Sodium benzoate monograph.* Retrieved from www.fao.org/ag/agn/jecfa-additives/specs/Monograph1/Additive-393.pdf

54. Eastman. (2013). *Product specification sheet for food grade sodium benzoate.* Retrieved from www.eastman.com/Supplemental/Unrestricted/35/SSG-32876.pdf

55. United States Food and Drug Administration. (2016). *Total diet study: factsheet for*

consumers. Available from www.fda.gov/Food/FoodScienceResearch/TotalDietStudy/ucm494299.htm

56. United States Food and Drug Administration. (2016). *Total diet study: elements results for market baskets 2006-2011..* Retrieved from www.fda.gov/downloads/Food/Food-ScienceResearch/TotalDietStudy/UCM184301.pdf

57. United States Food and Drug Administration. (2014). *What you need to know about mercury in fish and shellfish (brochure).* Retrieved from www.fda.gov/Food/Resources-ForYou/Consumers/ucm110591.htm

58. American Academy of Pediatrics. (2001). Technical report: mercury in the environment: implications for pediatricians. *Pediatrics,* 108:197. Retrieved from http://pediatrics.aappublications.org/content/pediatrics/108/1/197.full.pdf

59. Siddiqui, K., Bawazeer, N., & Joy, S.S. (2014). Variation in macro and trace elements in progression of type-2 diabetes. *Scientific World Journal,* 461591, 1-9. www.ncbi.nlm.nih.gov/pmc/articles/PMC4138889/pdf/TSWJ2014-461591.pdf

60. Foster, M., & Samman, S. (2010). Zinc and redox signaling: perturbations associated with cardiovascular disease and diabetes mellitus. *Antiox Redox Signal,* 13, 10, 1549-1573.

61. Malavolta, M., Giacconi, R., Piacenza, F., Santarelli, L., Cipriano, C., Costarelli, L., Tesei, S., Pierpaoli, S., Basso, A., Galeazzi, R., Lattanzio, F., & Mocchegiani, E. (2010). Plasma copper/zinc ratio: an inflammatory/nutritional biomarker as predictor of all-cause mortality in elderly population. *Biogerontology,* 11, 3, 309-319.

62. Federman, D.G., Kirsner, R.S., Federman, G.S. (1997). Pica: are you hungry for the facts? *Conn Med,* 61(4), 207-209.

63. Alabdali, A., Al-Ayadhi, L., & El-Ansary, A. (2014). A key role for an impaired detoxification mechanism in the etiology and severity of autism spectrum disorders. *Behavioral and Brain Functions,* 10:14. Retrieved from www.behavioralandbrainfunctions.com/content/10/1/14

64. Woo, H.D., Kim, D.W., Hong, Y-S., Kim, Y-M., Seo, J-H., Choe, B.M., Park, J.H., Kang, J-W., Yoo, J-H., Chueh, H.W., Lee, J.H., Kwak, M.J., & Kim, J. (2014). Dietary patterns in children with attention deficit/hyperactivity disorder (ADHD). *Nutrients,* 6, 1539-1553. Retrieved from www.ncbi.nlm.nih.gov/pmc/articles/PMC4011050/

CHAPTER 5

Recommended Videos

Dufault, R. (2014, April). The medicine of food. In J. Barreiro (Chair), *Patterns of health and wellbeing.* Symposium conducted at the Smithsonian Institute National Museum of the American Indian. Retrieved from www.youtube.com/watch?v=IwapwKitM0k

Lustig, R. (2009). *Sugar: the bitter truth.* Retrieved from www.youtube.com/watch?v=dBnniua6-oM

Spurlock, M. (2004). *Super size me.* Available on Netflix or Amazon.

References

1. Cordain L., Eaton S.B., Sebastian A., Mann N., Lindeberg S., Watkins B.A., O'Keefe J.H., & Brand-Miller J. (2005). Origins and evolution of the western diet: health implications for

the 21st century. *Am. J. Clin. Nutr,* 81, 341–354. Retrieved from http://ajcn .nutrition.org/content/81/2/341.full.pdf

2. Ruiz-Nunez, B., Pruimboom, L., Dijck-Brouwer, D.A.J., & Muskiet, F.A.J. (2013). Lifestyle and nutritional imbalances associated with western diseases: causes and consequences of chronic systemic low-grade inflammation in an evolutionary context. *Journal of Nutritional Biochemistry,* 24, 1183-1201. Retrieved from http://download.journals.elsevier-health.com/pdfs/journals/0955-2863/PIIS0955286313000545.pdf

3. Chilton, F.H., Murphy, R.C., Wilson, B.A., Sergeant, S., Ainsworth, H., Seeds, M.C., & Mathias, R.A. (2014). Diet-gene interactions and PUFA metabolism: a potential contributor to health disparities and human diseases. *Nutrients,* 6(5), 1993-2022. Retrieved from www.ncbi.nlm.nih.gov/pmc/articles/PMC4042578/pdf/nutrients-06-01993.pdf

4. Hawkes, C. (2006). Uneven dietary development: linking the policies and processes of globalization with the nutrition transition, obesity, and diet-related chronic diseases. *Global Health,* 2:4. Retrieved from www.ncbi.nlm.nih.gov/pmc/articles/PMC1440852/

5. Dufault, R., Schnoll, R., Lukiw, W.J., LeBlanc, B., Cornett, C., Patrick, L., Wallinga, D., Gilbert, S.G., & Crider, R. (2009). Mercury exposure, nutritional deficiencies and metabolic disruptions may affect learning in children. *Behavioral and Brain Functions,* 5:44. Retrieved from www.ncbi.nlm.nih.gov/pmc/articles/PMC2773803/#!po=76.0417

6. Zahniser, S., Kennedy, L., Nigatu, G., & McConnell, M. (2016). *A new outlook for the U.S.-Mexico sugar and sweetener market.* Retrieved from www.ers.usda.gov/webdocs/publications/sssm33501/60121_sssm-335-01.pdf?v=42593

7. Rivera, J.A., Barquera, S., Gonzalez-Cossio, T., Olaiz, G., & Sepulveda, J. (2004). Nutrition transition in Mexico and in other Latin American countries. *Nutrition Reviews,* 62(7 Pt 2):S149-157. Retrieved from www.researchgate.net/publication/229640567_Nutrition_Transition_in_Mexico_and_in_Other_Latin_American_Countries

8. Organization for Economic Co-operation and Development (OECD). (2014). *Obesity and the economics of prevention: fit not fat key facts—Mexico, update 2014.* Retrieved from www.oecd.org/mexico/Obesity-Update-2014-MEXICO_EN.pdf

9. Food and Agriculture Organization (FAO). (2013). *The state of food and agriculture,* pages 7 and 77. Retrieved from www.fao.org/docrep/018/i3300e/i3300e.pdf,

10. World Health Organization. (2014). *Mexico.* Retrieved from www.who.int/diabetes/country-profiles/mex_en.pdf?ua=1

11. ReportBuyer. (2014, February 10). *China edible vegetable oil industry report, 2013-2015.* Retrieved from www.prnewswire.com/news-releases/china-edible-vegetable-oil-industry-report-2013-2015-244719031.html

12. Ma, J. (2014, October 13). Blame for health crisis placed on poor knowledge. *South China Morning Post.* Retrieved from www.scmp.com/article/473991/blame-health-crisis-placed-poor-knowledge

13. Popkin, B.M. (2007). The world is fat. *Scientific American,* 88-95. Retrieved from http://sites.oxy.edu/clint/physio/article/worldisfat.pdf

14. World Health Organization. (2016). *Rate of diabetes in china "explosive."* Retrieved from www.wpro.who.int/china/mediacentre/releases/2016/20160406/en/

15. Gordon-Larsen, P., Wang, H., & Popkin, B.M. (2014). Overweight dynamics in Chinese

children and adults. *Obesity Reviews*, 15(01):37-48. Retrieved from www.ncbi.nlm.nih.gov/pmc/articles/PMC3951516/

16. Liberman, J.N., Berger, J.E., & Lewis, M. (2009). Prevalence of antihypertensive, antidiabetic, and dyslipidemic prescription medication use among children and adolescents. *Arch Pediatr Adolesc Med*, 163(4), 357-364.

17. Goran, M., Dumke, K., Bouret, S.G., Kayser, B., Walker, R.W., Blumberg, B. (2013). The obesogenic effect of high fructose exposure during early development. *Nat Rev Endocrinol*, 9(8), 494-500.

18. Vickers, M. H. (2014). Early life nutrition, epigenetics and programming of later life disease. *Nutrients*, 6, 2165-2178. Retrieved from www.ncbi.nlm.nih.gov/pmc/articles/PMC4073141/pdf/nutrients-06-02165.pdf

19. Stupin, J.H., & Arabin, B. (2014). Overweight and obesity before, during and after pregnancy. *Geburtshilfe Frauenheilkd*, 74(4), 639-645. Retrieved from www.ncbi.nlm.nih.gov/pmc/articles/PMC4119104/

20. Milne, D.B., & Nielsen, F.H. (2000). "The interaction between dietary fructose and magnesium adversely affects macromineral homeostasis in men." *J Am Coll Nutr*, 19, 31-37.

21. Ivaturi, R., & Kies, C. (1992). "Mineral balances in humans as affected by fructose, high-fructose corn syrup, and sucrose." *Plant Foods for Hum Nutr*, 42(2), 143-151.

22. Ward, N.I., Soulsbury, K., Zettel, V.H., Colquhoun, I.D., Bunday, S., & Barnes, B. (1990). The influence of the chemical additive tartrazine on the zinc status of hyperactive children-a double-blind placebo-controlled study. *J Nutr Med*, 1, 51–57.

23. Laks, D.R. (2009). Assessment of chronic mercury exposure in the U.S. population, national health and nutrition examination survey, 1999-2006. *Biometals*, 22(6), 1103-14.

24. Ettinger, A.S., Bovet, P., Plange-Rhule, J., Forrester, T.E., Lambert, E.V., Lupoli, N., Shine, J., Dugas, L.R., Shoham, D., Durazo-Arvizu, R.A., Cooper, R.S., Luke, A. (2014). Distribution of metals exposure and associations with cardiometabolic risk factors in the "Modeling the Epidemiologic Transition Study". *Environmental Health*, 13:90. Retrieved from www.ncbi.nlm.nih.gov/pmc/articles/PMC4240881/

25. Eom, S.Y., Choi, S.H., Ahn, S.J., Kim, D.K., Kim,D.W., Lim, J.A., Choi, B.S., Shin, H.J., Yun, S.W., Yoon, H.J., Kim, Y.M., Hong, Y.S., Yun, Y.W., Sohn, S.J., Kim, H., Park, K.S., Pyo, H.S., Kim, H., Oh, S.Y., Kim, J., Lee, S.A., Ha, M., Kwon, H.J., Park, J.D. (2014). Reference levels of blood mercury and association with metabolic syndrome in Korean adults. *International Archives of Occupational and Environmental Health*,87(5), 501-13.

26. He, K., Xun, P., Liu, K., Morris, S., Reis, J., Guallar, E. (2013). Mercury exposure in young adulthood and incidence of diabetes later in life: the CARDIA Trace Element Study. *Diabetes Care*, 36(6), 1584-9. Retrieved from www.ncbi.nlm.nih.gov/pmc/articles/PMC3661833/

27. Chang, J.W., Chen, H.L., Su, H.J., Liao, P.C., Guo, H.R., Lee, C.C. (2011). Simultaneous exposure of non-diabetics to high levels of dioxins and mercury increases their risk of insulin resistance. *Journal of Hazardous Materials*. 185(2-3), 749-55.

28. Solenkova, N.V., Newman, J.D., Berger, J.S., Thurston, G., Hochman, J.S., Lamas, G.A. (2014). Metal pollutants and cardiovascular disease: mechanisms and consequences of exposure. *Am Heart J*, 168(6), 812-22. Retrieved from www.ahjonline.com/article/S0002-8703%2814%2900426-8/abstract?cc=y

29. Wildemann, T.M., Weber, L.P., Siciliano, S.D. (2014). Combined exposure to lead, inorganic mercury and methylmercury shows deviation from additivity for cardiovascular toxicity in rats. *J Appl Toxicol*, 35(8), 918-926.

30. Dufault, R., Berg, Z., Crider, R., Schnoll, R., Wetsit, L., Two Bulls, W., Gilbert, S.G., Kingston, H.M. "Skip," Wolle, M.M., Rahman, G.M.M., Laks, D.R. (2015). Blood inorganic mercury is directly associated with glucose levels in the human population and may be linked to processed food intake. *Integrative Molecular Medicine*, 2(3), 181-194. Retrieved from http://oatext.com/pdf/IMM-2-134.pdf

31. Centers for Disease Control and Prevention. (2015). *About the national health and nutrition examination survey.* Retrieved from www.cdc.gov/nchs/nhanes/about_nhanes.htm

32. Thirumoorthy, N., Sunder, A.S., Kumar, K.T.M., Kumar, M.S., Ganesh, G.N.K., & Chatterjee, M. (2011). A review of metallothionein isoforms and their role in pathophysiology. *World Journal of Surgical Oncology*, 9:54. Retrieved from www.ncbi.nlm.nih.gov/pmc/articles/PMC3114003/pdf/1477-7819-9-54.pdf

33. National Institutes of Health. (2014). *Magnesium fact sheet for health professionals.* Retrieved from http://ods.od.nih.gov/factsheets/Magnesium-HealthProfessional/

34. Konikowska, K., Regulska-Ilow, B., & Rozanska, D. (2012). The influence of components of diet on the symptoms of ADHD in children. *Rocz Panstw Zakl Hig*, 63(2), 127-134.

35. United States Department of Agriculture. (2009). *What we eat in America, NHANES 2005-2006.* Retrieved from www.ars.usda.gov/SP2UserFiles/Place/12355000/pdf/0506/usual_nutrient_intake_vitD_ca_phos_mg_2005-06.pdf

36. Centers for Disease Control and Prevention. (2008). *Nutrition and the health of young people.* Retrieved from www.cdc.gov/HealthyYouth/nutrition/pdf/facts.pdf

37. Elizabeth, K.E., Krishnan, V., & Vijayakumar, T. (2008). Umbilical cord blood nutrients in low birth weight babies in relation to birth weight & gestational age. *Indian J Med Res*, 128(2), 128-133.

38. Hovdenak, N., & Haram, K. (2012). Influence of mineral and vitamin supplements on pregnancy outcome. *Eur J Obstet Gynecol Reprod Biol*, 164(2), 127-132.

39. Singh, G.K., Kenney, M.K., Ghandour, R.M., Kogan, M.D., & Lu, M.C. (2013). Mental health outcomes in US children and adolescents born prematurely or with low birthweight. *Depress Res Treat*, 570743. Retrieved from www.ncbi.nlm.nih.gov/pmc/articles/PMC3845867/

40. Maramara, L.A., He, W., & Ming, X. (2014). Pre- and perinatal risk factors for autism spectrum disorder in a New Jersey cohort. *J Child Neurol*. 29(12), 1645-1651.

41. Pettersson, E., Sjolander, A., Almqvist, C., Anckarsater, H., D'Onofrio, B.M., Lichtenstein, P., & Larsson, H. (2014). Birth weight as an independent predictor of ADHD symptoms: a within-twin pair analysis. *J Child Psychol Psychiatry*. 56(4), 453-459.

42. Centers for Disease Control and Prevention. (2014). *Lead.* Retrieved from www.cdc.gov/nceh/lead/

43. Bruening, K., Kemp, F.W., Simone, N., Holding, Y., Louria, D.B., & Bogden, J.D. (1999). Dietary calcium intakes of urban children at risk of lead poisoning. *Environmental Health*

Perspectives, 107(6), 431-435. Retrieved from www.ncbi.nlm.nih.gov/pmc/articles/PMC1566572/pdf/envhper00511-0047.pdf

44.Mahaffey, K.R., Gartside, P.S., & Glueck, C.J. (1986). "Blood lead levels and dietary calcium intake in 1 to 11 year-old children: the second national health and nutrition examination survey," 1976 to 1980. *Pediatrics ,* 78, 257-262.

45. Shannon, M., & Graef, J.W. (1996). Lead intoxication in children with pervasive developmental disorders. *J Toxicol Clin Toxicol,* 34, 177-181.

46. Eubig, P.A., Aguiar, A., & Schantz, S.L. (2010). "Lead and PCBs as risk factors for attention deficit/hyperactivity disorder." *Environ Health Perspect,* 118, 1654-1667. Retrieved from www.ncbi.nlm.nih.gov/pmc/articles/PMC3002184/

47. United States Department of Agriculture. (2014). *Food availability (per capita) data system.* Retrieved from www.ers.usda.gov/data-products/food-availability-%28per-capita%29-data-system.aspx#.VBNJ2KOJWUR

48. Takaya, J., Iharada, A., Okihana, H., & Kaneko, K. (2013). A calcium-deficient diet in pregnant, nursing rats induces hypomethylation of specific cytosines in the 11b-hydroxysteroid dehydrogenase-1 promoter in pup liver. *Nutr Res,* 33(1), 961-970.

49. Obeid, R. (2013). The metabolic burden of methyl donor deficiency with focus on the betaine homocysteine methyltransferase pathway. *Nutrients,* 5, 3481-3495. Retrieved from www.ncbi.nlm.nih.gov/pmc/articles/PMC3798916/pdf/nutrients-05-03481.pdf

50. James, S.J., Melnyk, S., Jernigan, S., Hubanks, A., Rose, S., & Gaylor, D.W. (2008). Abnormal transmethylation/transsulfuration metabolism and DNA hypomethylation among parents of children with autism. *J Autism Dev Disord,* 38(10), 1966-1975. Retrieved from www.ncbi.nlm.nih.gov/pmc/articles/PMC2584168/

51. Kim, G.H., Ryan, J.J., Archer, S.L. (2013). The role of redox signaling in epigenetics and cardiovascular disease. *Antioxid Redox Signal,* 18(15), 1920-1936. Retrieved from www.ncbi.nlm.nih.gov/pmc/articles/PMC3624767/

52. Luttmer, R, Spijkerman, A.M., Kok, R.M., Jakobs, C., Blom, H.J., Serne, E.H., Dekker, J. & M., Smulders, Y.M. (2013). Metabolic syndrome components are associated with DNA hypomethylation. *Obes Res Clin Pract,* 7(2), e106-e115.

53. Carlin, J., George, R., & Reyes, T.M. (2013). Methyl donor supplementation blocks the adverse effects of maternal high fat diet on offspring physiology. *PLOS ONE,* 8(5), e63549. Retrieved from www.ncbi.nlm.nih.gov/pmc/articles/PMC3642194/pdf/pone.0063549.pdf

54. Drummond, E.M., & Gibney, E.R. (2013). Epigenetic regulation in obesity. *Curr Opin Clin Nutr Metab Care,* 16(4), 392-397.

CHAPTER 6

Recommended Videos

Institute for Agriculture and Trade Policy (2012). *The autism revolution: thinking about environment and food.* Retrieved from www.youtube.com/watch?v=mgAsDXgo5ao

References

1. Centers for Disease Control and Prevention. (2016). *Autism and developmental disabilities monitoring network (ADDM).* Retrieved from www.cdc.gov/ncbddd/autism/addm.html

2. American Psychological Association. (2016). *Autism.* Retrieved from www.apa.org/topics/autism/index.aspx

3. Dufault, R., Lukiw, W.J., Crider, R., Schnoll, R., Wallinga, D., & Deth, R. (2012). A macroepigenetic approach to identify the factors responsible for the autism epidemic in the United States. *Clinical Epigenetics,* 4:6. Retrieved from www.clinicalepigeneticsjournal.com/content/4/1/6

4. American Psychological Association. (2016). *ADHD.* www.apa.org/topics/adhd/

5. Visser, S.N., et al. (2014). Key findings: trends in parent-report of health care provider-diagnosis and medication treatment for ADHD: United States, 2003-2011. *Journal of American Academy of Child and Adolescent Psychiatry,* 53(1):34-46. Retrieved from www.jaacap.com/article/S0890-8567(13)00594-7/pdf

6. Centers for Disease Control and Prevention. (2016). *Attention deficit hyperactivity disorder (ADHD): data and statistics.* Retrieved from www.cdc.gov/ncbddd/adhd/data.html

7. PubMed.gov (2016). *Search for etiology of autism.* Retrieved from www.ncbi.nlm.nih.gov/pubmed/?term=autism+and+etiology

8. PubMed.gov (2016). *Search for etiology of ADHD.* Retrieved from www.ncbi.nlm.nih.gov/pubmed/?term=ADHD+and+etiology

9. Palmer, R.F., Blanchard, S., Stein, Z., Mandell, D., & Miller, C. (2006). Environmental mercury release, special education rates, and autism disorder: an ecological study of Texas. *Health Place,* 12(2):203-209.

10. Sathyanarayana Rao, T.S., & Andrade, C. (2011). The MMR vaccine and autism: sensation, refutation, retraction, and fraud. *Indian Journal of Psychiatry,* 53(2):95-96. Retrieved from www.ncbi.nlm.nih.gov/pmc/articles/PMC3136032/

11. SafeMinds. (2016). *Leadership.* Retrieved from www.safeminds.org/about-2/executive-board/

12. Bernard, S., Enayati, A., Redgrave, L., Roger, H., & Binstock, T. (2001). Autism: a novel form of mercury poisoning. *Medical Hypothesis,* 56(4):462-471.

13. SafeMinds. (2016). *Our peer reviewed publications.* Retrieved from www.safeminds.org/wp-content/uploads/2013/04/SafeMinds-research-publications-2000-2013-with-intro-FINAL.pdf

14. SafeMinds. (2010). *Mercury in vaccines.* Retrieved from www.safeminds.org/wp-content/uploads/2013/04/mercury_in-vaccines.pdf

15. United States Food and Drug Administration. (2015). *Thimerosal in vaccines.* Retrieved from www.fda.gov/BiologicsBloodVaccines/SafetyAvailability/VaccineSafety/ucm096228.htm

16. United States Centers for Disease Control. (2015). *Autism spectrum disorder: data & statistics.* Retrieved from www.cdc.gov/ncbddd/autism/data.html

17. United States Centers for Disease Control. (2015). *Vaccines do not cause autism.* Retrieved from www.cdc.gov/vaccinesafety/concerns/autism.html

18. Murch, S.H., Anthony, A., Casson, D.H., Malik, M., Berelowitz, M., Dhillon, A.P., Thomson, M.A., Valentine, A., Davies, S.E., & Walker-Smith, J.A. (2004). Retraction of an interpretation. *Lancet,* volume 363:750.

19. Burns, J. F. (2010, May 24). British medical council bars doctor who linked vaccine with autism. *New York Times.* Retrieved from www.nytimes.com/2010/05/25/health/policy/25autism.html

20. Generation Rescue. (2016). *Background.* Retrieved from http://generationrescue.org/about/background/

21. Generation Rescue. (2016). *Resources.* Retrieved from http://generationrescue.org/resources/

22. Generation Rescue. (2016). *Applying for the rescue family grant.* Retrieved from https://generationrescue.org/member-log-in/join-grant/

23. National Vaccine Information Center. (2016). *About national vaccine information center.* Retrieved from www.nvic.org/about.aspx

24. National Vaccine Information Center. (2016). *The moral right to conscientious, philosophical and personal belief exemption to vaccination.* Retrieved from www.nvic.org/informed-consent.aspx

25. Bouchard, M.F., Bellinger, D.C., Wright, R.O., Weisskopf, M.G. (2010). Attention-deficit hyperactivity disorder and urinary metabolites of organophosphate pesticides. *Pediatric,* 125, e1270-e1277. Retrieved from http://pediatrics.aappublications.org/content/125/6/e1270.full.pdf+html

26. Shelton, J.F., Geraghty, E.M., Tancredi, D.J., Delwiche, L.D., Schmidt, B.R., Hansen, R.L., Hertz-Picciotto, I. (2014). Neurodevelopmental disorders and prenatal residential proximity to agricultural pesticides: the CHARGE study. *Environmental Health Perspectives,* 122(10), 1103-1109. Retrieved from www.ncbi.nlm.nih.gov/pmc/articles/PMC4181917/pdf/ehp.1307044.pdf

27. Nevison, C.D. (2014). A comparison of temporal trends in the united states autism prevalence to trends in suspected environmental factors. *Environmental Health,* 13:73. Retrieved from www.ncbi.nlm.nih.gov/pmc/articles/PMC4177682/pdf/12940_2014_Article_781.pdf

28. Holzman, D. (2014). Pesticides and autism spectrum disorders. *Environmental Health Perspectives,* 122(10), A280. Retrieved from www.ncbi.nlm.nih.gov/pmc/articles/PMC4181911/pdf/ehp.122-A280.pdf

29. Bjorling-Poulsen, M., Andersen, H.R., Grandjean, P. (2008). Potential developmental neurotoxicity of pesticides used in Europe. *Environmental Health,* 7:50. www.ehjournal.net/content/7/1/50

30. Harari, R., Julvez, J., Murata, K., Barr, D., Bellinger, D.C., Debes, F., Grandjean, P. (2010). Neurobehavioral deficits and increased blood pressure in school-age children prenatally exposed to pesticides. *Environmental Health Perspectives* 118, 890-6. Retrieved from www.ncbi.nlm.nih.gov/pmc/articles/PMC2898869/pdf/ehp-118-890.pdf

31. Jurewicz, J. & Hanke, W. (2008).Prenatal and childhood exposure to pesticides and neurobehavioral development: review of epidemiological studies. *International Journal of Occupational Medicine and Environmental Health* 21, 121-32.

32. Bouchard, M.F., Chevrier, J., Harley, K.G., Kogut, K., Vedar, M., Calderon, N., Trujillo, C., Johnson, C., Bradman, A., Barr, D.B., Eskenazi, B. (2011). Prenatal exposure to organophosphate pesticides and IQ in 7-year-old children. *Environmental Health Perspectives*, 119, 1189-95. Retrieved from www.ncbi.nlm.nih.gov/pmc/articles/PMC3237357/pdf/ehp.1003185.pdf

33. Patel, K., Luke, C. T. (2007). A comprehensive approach to treating autism and attention-deficit-hyperactivity-disorder: a prepilot study. *Journal of Alternative and Complementary Medicine*, 13(10), 1091-1097.

34. Pellow, J., Solomon, E.M., Barnard, C.N. Complementary and alternative medical therapies for children with attention-deficit/hyperactivity disorder (ADHD). *Alternative Medicine Review*, 16(4), 323-337. www.altmedrev.com/publications/16/4/323.pdf

35. Lu, C., Toepel, K., Irish, R., Fenske, R.A., Barr, D.B., Bravo, R. (2006). Organic diets significantly lower children's dietary exposure to organophosphorus pesticides. *Environmental Health Perspectives*, 114(2), 260-263. Retrieved from www.ncbi.nlm.nih.gov/pmc/articles/PMC1367841/pdf/ehp0114-000260.pdf

36. Costa, L.G., Giordano, G., Furlong, C.E. (2011). Pharmacological and dietary modulators of paraoxonase 1 (PON1) activity and expression: the hunt goes on. *Biochem Pharmacol*, 81(3), 337-344. Retrieved from www.ncbi.nlm.nih.gov/pmc/articles/PMC3077125/pdf/nihms253678.pdf

37. University of Florida. (2015). *Pesticide toxicity profile: carbamate pesticides.* Retrieved from http://edis.ifas.ufl.edu/pi088

38. Delaware Health and Social Services. (2015), *Organophosphate and carbamate pesticides.* Retrieved from http://dhss.delaware.gov/dhss/dph/files/organophospestfaq.pdf

39. Milne, D.B., & Nielsen, F.H. (2000). The interaction between dietary fructose and magnesium adversely affects macromineral homeostasis in men. *J Am Coll Nutr*, 19, 31-37.

40. Pasca, S.P., Dronca, E., Nemes, B., Kaucsar T., Endreffy, E., Iftene, F., Benga, I, Cornean, R., Dronca, M. (2010). Paraoxonase 1 activities and polymorphisms in autism spectrum disorders. *J Cell Mol Med*, 14(3), 600-607. Retrieved from www.ncbi.nlm.nih.gov/pmc/articles/PMC3823459/pdf/jcmm0014-0600.pdf

41. Ceylan, M.F., Sener, S., Bayraktar, A.C., Kavutcu, M. (2012). Changes in oxidative stress and cellular immunity serum markers in attention-deficit/hyperactivity disorder. *Psychiatry and Clinical Neurosciences*, 66, 220-226. Retrieved from http://onlinelibrary.wiley.com/doi/10.1111/j.1440-1819.2012.02330.x/pdf

42. Fortenberry, G.Z., et al. (2014). Paraoxonase 1 polymorphisms and attention/hyperactivity in school-age children from Mexico City, Mexico. *Environmental Research*, 132:342-349.

43. Costa, L.G., Vitalone, A., Cole, T.B., Furlong, C.E. (2005). Modulation of paraoxonase (PON1) activity. *Biochem Pharmacol*, 69, 541-550.

44. Laks, D.R. (2009). Assessment of chronic mercury exposure within the U.S. population, National Health and Nutrition Examination Survey, 1999-2006. *Biometals*, 22(6), 1103-1114.

45. Huen, K., Harley, K., Bradman, A., Eskenazi, B., Holland, N. (2010). Longitudinal changes in PON1 enzymatic activities in mexican-american mothers and children with different genotypes and halotypes. *Toxicol Appl Pharmacol*, 244, 181-189.

46. Eskenazi, B., Huen, K., Marks, A., Harley, K.G., Bradman, A., Barr, D.B., Holland, N. (2010). PON1 and neurodevelopment in children from the CHAMACOS study exposed to organophosphate pesticides *in utero*. *Environmental Health Perspectives*, 118, 1775-1781. Retrieved from www.ncbi.nlm.nih.gov/pmc/articles/PMC3002199/pdf/ehp-118-1775.pdf

47. Li, W.F., Pan, M.H., Chung, M.C., Ho, C.K., Chuang, H.Y. (2006). Lead exposure is associated with decreased paraoxonase 1 (PON1) activity and genotypes. *Environmental Health Perspectives*, 114(8), 1233-1236. Retrieved from www.ncbi.nlm.nih.gov/pmc/articles/PMC1552024/pdf/ehp0114-001233.pdf

48. Kamal, M., Fathy, M.M., Taher, E., Hasan, M., Tolba, M. (2011). Assessment of the role of paraoxonase gene polymorphism (Q192R) and paraoxonase activity in the susceptibility to atherosclerosis among lead-exposed workers. *Ann Saudi Med*, 31(5), 481-487. Retrieved from www.ncbi.nlm.nih.gov/pmc/articles/PMC3183682/

49. Lacasana, M., Lopez-Flores, I., Rodriguez-Barranco, M., Aguilar-Garduno, C., Blanco-Munoz, J., Perez-Mendez, O., Gonzales-Alzaga, B., Bassol, S., Cebrian, M.E. (2010). Interaction between organophosphate pesticide exposure and PON1 activity on thyroid function. *Toxicol Appl Pharmacol*, 249(1), 16-24.

50. Detweiler, M.B. (2014). Organophosphate intermediate syndrome with neurological complications of extrapyramidla symptoms in clinical practice. *J Neurosci Rural Prac*, 5(3), 298-301. Retrieved from www.ncbi.nlm.nih.gov/pmc/articles/PMC4078626/

51. Kellman, R. (2011). The thyroid-autism connection: the role of endocrine disruptors. *Journal of Autism One*, 2, 111-117. Retrieved from http://nancymullanmd.com/pdf/The ThyroidAutismConnection.pdf

52. Rossett, R., Surowska, A., & Tappy, L. (2016). Pathogenesis of cardiovascular and metabolic diseases: are fructose-containing sugars more involved than other dietary calories? *Current Hypertension Reports*, 18:44. Retrieved from www.ncbi.nlm.nih.gov/pmc/articles/PMC4850171/pdf/11906_2016_Article_652.pdf

53. Rivera, H.M., Christiansen, K.J., & Sullivan, E.L. (2015). The role of maternal obesity in the risk of neuropsychiatric disorders. *Frontiers in Neuroscience*, 9:194. Retrieved from www.ncbi.nlm.nih.gov/pmc/articles/PMC4471351/pdf/fnins-09-00194.pdf

54. Pugh, S.J. et al. (2016). Gestational weight gain, prepregnancy body mass index and offspring attention-deficit hyperactivity disorder symptoms and behavior at age 10. BLOG, doi. 10.1111/1471-0528.13909

55. Li, M. et al. (2016). The association of maternal obesity and diabetes with autism and other developmental disabilities. *Pediatrics*, 137(2):e20152206.

56. Nahum, S.K. et al. (2016). Prenatal exposure to gestational diabetes mellitus as an independent risk factor for long-term neuropsychiatric morbidity of the offspring. *American Journal of Obstetrics and Gynecology*, 215(3):380.e1-7.

57. Dufault, R., Schnoll, R., Lukiw, W.J., LeBlanc, B., Cornett, C., Patrick, L., Wallinga, D., Gilbert, S.G., & Crider, R. (2009). Mercury exposure, nutritional deficiencies and metabolic disruptions may affect learning in children. *Behavioral and Brain Functions*, 5:44. Retrieved from http://behavioralandbrainfunctions.biomedcentral.com/articles/10.1186/1744-9081-5-44

58. Saad, A.F. et al. (2016). High-fructose diet in pregnancy leads to fetal programming of

hypertension, insulin resistance, and obesity in adult offspring. *American Journal of Obstetrics and Gynecology,* 215(3):e1-6.

59. Rossiter, M.D., Colapinto, C.K., Khan, M.K., McIsaac, J.L., Williams, P.L., Kirk, S.F., Veugelers, P.J. (2015). Breast, formula and combination feeding in relation to childhood obesity in Nova Scotia, Canada. *Matern Child Health J,* Feb. 6.

60. Oddy, W.H., Mori, T.A., Huang, R.C., Marsh, J.A., Pennell, C.E., Chivers, P.T., Hands, B.P., Jacoby, P., Rzehak, P., Koletzko, B.V., Beilin, L.J. (2014). Early infant feeding and diposity risk: from infancy to adulthood. *Ann Nutr Metab,* 64(3-4), 262-70.

61. Lumeng, J.C., Taveras, E.M., Birch, L., Yanovski, S.Z. (2015). Prevention of obesity in infancy and early childhood: a national institutes of health workshop. *JAMA Pediatr,* 169(5), 484-490.

62. Schultz, S.T., et al. (2006). Breastfeeding, infant formula supplementation, and autistic disorder: the results of a parent survey. *International Breastfeeding Journal,* 1:16. Retrieved from www.ncbi.nlm.nih.gov/pmc/articles/PMC1578554/pdf/1746-4358-1-16.pdf

63. Salhia, H.O., Al-Nasser, L.A., Taher, L.S., Al-Khatbaami, A.M. (2014). Systemic review of the epidemiology of autism in Arab Gulf countries. *Neuroscience,* 19(4):291-296. Retrieved from www.ncbi.nlm.nih.gov/pmc/articles/PMC4727667/pdf/Neurosciences-19-291.pdf

64. Cruz, G.C., Din, Z., Feri, C.D., Balaoing, A.M., Gonzales, E.M., Navidad, H.M., Schlaaff, M.F., Winter, J. (2009). Analysis of toxic heavy metals (arsenic, lead, and mercury) in selected infant formula milk commercially available in the Philippines by AAS. *E-International Scientific Research Journal,* 1(1), 40-50.

65. Abuzariba, S.M., Gazette, M. (2015). Heavy metals in selected infant milk formula. *World Academy of Science, Engineering and Technology,* 2(2). Abstract available at www.waset.org/abstracts/18908

66. Pandelova, M., Lopez, W.L., Michalke, B., Schramm, K-W. (2012). Ca, cd, cu, fe, hg, mn, ni, pb, se, and zn contents in baby foods from the EU market: comparison of assessed infant intakes with the present safety limits for minerals and trace elements. *Journal of Food Composition and Analysis,* 27, 120-127.

67. Dabeka, R.W., McKenzie, A.D. (2012). Survey of total mercury in infant formulae and oral electrolytes sold in Canada. *Food Addit Contam Part B Surveil,* 5(1), 65-9.

68. Vela, N.P., Heitkemper, D.T. (2004). Total arsenic determination and speciation in infant food products by ion chromatography-inductively coupled plasma-mass spectrometry. *J AOAC Int,* 87(1), 244-52.

69. Martins, C., Vasco, E., Paixao, E., Alvito, P. (2013). Total mercury in infant food, occurrence and exposure assessment in Portugal. *Food Addit Contam Part B Surveil,* 6(3), 151-7.

70. Shafai, T., Mustafa, M., Hild, T., Mulari, J., Curtis, A. (2014). The association of early weaning and formula feeding in autism spectrum disorders. *Breastfeeding Medicine,* 9(5), 275-276.

71. Sabuncuoglu, O., Orengul, C., Bikmazer, A., Kaynar, S.Y. (2014). Breastfeeding and parafunctional oral habits in children with and without attention-deficit/hyperactivity disorder. *Breastfeed Med,* 9(5), 244-50.

72. Zhou, F., et al. (2016). Dietary, nutrient patterns and blood essential elements in

Chinese children with ADHD. Nutrients, 8(6). Retrieved from www.ncbi.nlm.nih.gov/pmc/articles/PMC4924193/pdf/nutrients-08-00352.pdf

73. Ward, N. (1997). Assessment of chemical factors in relation to child hyperactivity. *J Nutr Environ Med*, 7:333-342.

74. Ward, N.I., Soulsbury, K.A., Zettel, V.H., Colquhoun, I.D., Bunday, S., & Barnes, B. (1990). The influence of the chemical additive tartrazine on the zinc status of hyperactive children-a double-blind placebo controlled study. *J Nutr Med* 1990, 1(1), 51-57.

75. Bateman, B., Warner, J.O., Hutchinson, E., Dean, T., Rowlandson, P., Gant, C., Grundy, J., Fitzgerald, C., & Stevenson, J. (2004). The effects of a double blind, placebo controlled artificial food colorings and sodium benzoate preservative challenge on hyperactivity in a general population sample of preschool children. *Arch Dis Child*, 89, 506-511. Retrieved from www.ncbi.nlm.nih.gov/pmc/articles/PMC1719942/pdf/v089p00506.pdf

76. McCann Food additives and hyperactive behavior in 3-year-old and 8/9-year-old children in the community: a randomized, double-blinded placebo-controlled trial. *Lancet* 2007, 370(9598), 1560-1567. www.feingold.org/Research/PDFstudies/Stevenson2007.pdf

77. Konikowska, K., Regulska-Ilow, B., & Rozanska, D. (2012). The influence of components of diet on the symptoms of ADHD in children. *Rocz Panstw Zakl Hig*, 63(2), 127-134.

78. Adams, K. M., Kohlmeier, M., & Zeisel, S. H. (2010). Nutrition education in U.S. medical schools: Latest update of a national survey. *Academic Medicine*, 85(9), 1537-1542. doi:10.1097/ACM.0b013e3181eab71b

79. Frantz, D. J., Munroe, C., McClave, S. A., & Martindale, R. (2011). Current perception of nutrition education in U.S. medical schools. *Current Gastroenterology Reports*, 13(4), 376-379. doi:10.1007/s11894-011-0202-z

80. United States Food and Drug Administration. (2013). *Medication guide: Ritalin*. Retrieved from www.fda.gov/downloads/Drugs/DrugSafety/ucm089090.pdf

81. Centers for Disease Control and Prevention. (2016). *Autism spectrum disorder: data and statistics.* Retrieved from www.cdc.gov/ncbddd/autism/data.html

82. Leigh, J.P., & Du, J. (2015). Brief report: forecasting the economic burden of autism in 2015 and 2025 in the United States. *Journal of Autism and Developmental Disorders*, 45(12):4135-4139.

83. Pelham, W.E., Foster, E.M., & Robb, J.A. (2007). The economic impact of attention deficit/hyperactivity disorder in children and adolescents. *Journal of Pediatric Psychology*, 32(6):711-727. Retrieved from http://jpepsy.oxfordjournals.org/content/32/6/711.long

84. Dall, T.M., Yang, W., Halder, P., Pang, B., Massoudi, M., Wintfeld, N., Semilla, A.P., Franz, J., & Hogan, P.F. (2014). The economic burden of elevated blood glucose levels in 2012: diagnosed and undiagnosed diabetes, gestational diabetes mellitus, and prediabetes. *Diabetes Care*, 37(12):3172-3179. Retrieved from http://care.diabetesjournals.org/content/37/12/3172

85. Crider, K.S., Yang, T.P., Berry, R.J., & Bailey, L.B. (2012). Folate and DNA methylation: a review of molecular mechanisms and the evidence for folate's role. *Advances in Nutrition*, 3, 21-38. Retrieved from http://advances.nutrition.org/content/3/1/21.full.pdf+html

86. LaSalle, J. (2011). A genomic point-of-view on environmental factors influencing the

human brain methylome. *Epigenetics,* 6(7), 862- 869. Retrieved from www.ncbi.nlm .nih.gov/pmc/articles/PMC3154427/pdf/epi0607_0862.pdf

CHAPTER 7

1. Food and Drug Administration. (2015). *When and why was FDA formed?*Retrieved from www.fda.gov/AboutFDA/Transparency/Basics/ucm214403.htm

2. Food and Drug Administration. (2009). *FDA history: part I.* Retrieved from www.fda.gov/AboutFDA/WhatWeDo/History/Origin/ucm054819.htm

3. Gandhi, L. (2013, August 26). A history of snake oil salesmen. *NPR,* Retrieved from www.npr.org/sections/codeswitch/2013/08/26/215761377/a-history-of-snake-oil-sales-men

4. Tirumalai, G., Long, A. (2013). *United States pharmacopeial convention: respecting the past, moving confidently into the future.* Retrieved from www.usp.org/sites/default/files/ usp_pdf/EN/aboutUSP/usp_history_final_with_acknowledgement.pdf

5. U.S. Pharmacopeial Convention. (2015). *About USP.* Retrieved from www.usp .org/about-usp

6. Food and Drug Administration. (2016). *What does FDA do?*Retrieved from www.fda.gov/AboutFDA/Transparency/Basics/ucm194877.htm

7. Janssen, W.F. (1981). The story of the laws behind the labels. *FDA Consumer.* www.fda.gov/AboutFDA/WhatWeDo/History/Overviews/ucm056044.htm

8. Food and Drug Administration. (2015). *History of the GRAS list and SCOGS review.* Retrieved from www.fda.gov/food/ingredientspackaginglabeling/gras/scogs/ucm 084142.htm

9. FDA Direct Food Substance Affirmed as Generally Recognized as Safe; High Fructose Corn Syrup, 21 CFR Parts 182 and 184. (1996). Retrieved from http://sweet surprise.com/sites/default/files/pdf/HFCS_GRAS_8-23-1996.pdf

10. Food and Drug Administration. (2015). *GRAS substances (SCOGS) database.* Retrieved from www.fda.gov/Food/IngredientsPackagingLabeling/GRAS/SCOGS/ucm2006852 .htm

11. Food and Drug Administration. (2013). *Food labeling guide.* Retrieved from www.fda.gov/Food/GuidanceRegulation/GuidanceDocumentsRegulatoryInforma-tion/LabelingNutrition/ucm2006828.htm#background

12. Food and Drug Administration. (2013). *Guidance for industry: a food labeling guide (6. Ingredient lists).* Retrieved from www.fda.gov/Food/GuidanceRegulation/GuidanceDoc-umentsRegulatoryInformation/LabelingNutrition/ucm064880.htm#preservatives

13. Food and Drug Administration. (2013). *Guidance for industry: a food labeling guide (6. Ingredient lists). On trace amount.* Retrieved from www.fda.gov/Food/GuidanceRegula-tion/GuidanceDocumentsRegulatoryInformation/LabelingNutrition/ucm064880.htm# declare

14. Food and Drug Administration. (2016). *"Natural" on food labeling.* Retrieved from www.fda.gov/Food/GuidanceRegulation/GuidanceDocumentsRegulatoryInforma-tion/LabelingNutrition/ucm456090.htm

15. Food and Drug Administration. (2010). *Open letter to industry from Dr. Hamburg.* Retrieved from www.fda.gov/Food/IngredientsPackagingLabeling/LabelingNutrition/ucm202733.htm

16. Celiac Disease Foundation. (2015). *What is gluten?*Retrieved from http://celiac.org/live-gluten-free/glutenfreediet/what-is-gluten/

17. Food and Drug Administration. (2015). *Questions and answers: gluten-free food labeling rule.* Retrieved from www.fda.gov/food/guidanceregulation/guidancedocumentsregulatoryinformation/allergens/ucm362880.htm

18. Kim, H., Patel, K., & Orosz, E. (2016). Time trends in the prevalence of celiac disease and gluten-free diet in the US population. *JAMA Internal Medicine*, 176(11): 1716-1717.

19. Puglise, N. (2016). More Americans are eating gluten-free despite not having celiac disease. *The Guardian.* Retrieved from https://www.theguardian.com/society/2016/sep/06/gluten-free-eating-celiac-disease-marketing-trend-diet.

20. Stevens, L., & Rashid, M. (2008). Gluten-free and regular foods: a cost comparison. *Canadian Journal of Dietetic Practice and Research*, 69(3): 147–150.

21. Strom, S. (2014, February 17). A big bet on gluten-free. *The New York Times.* Retrieved from www.nytimes.com/2014/02/18/business/food-industry-wagers-big-on-gluten-free.html?_r=0

22. Barack, L. (2011, August 19). Food giants mine the gluten-free gold rush. *Fortune.* Retrieved from www.nytimes.com/2014/02/18/business/food-industry-wagers-big-on-gluten-free.html?_r=0

23. Mintel. (2015). *Half of Americans think gluten-free diets are a fad while 25% eat gluten-free foods.* Retrieved from www.mintel.com/press-centre/food-and-drink/half-of-americans-think-gluten-free-diets-are-a-fad-while-25-eat-gluten-free-foods

24. GF & AF Expo. (2015). *Our mission.* Retrieved from http://gfafexpo.com/about-us/

25. Wu, J.H., Neal, B., Trevena, H., Crino, M., Stuart-Smith, W., Faulkner-Hogg, K., Yu, L., Dunford, E. (2015). Are gluten-free foods healthier than non-gluten-free foods? An evaluation of supermarket products in Australia. *Br J Nutr,* 1-7 [Epub ahead of print].

26. Stewart, P.A., Hyman, S.L., Schmidt, B.L., Macklin, E.A., Reynolds, A., Johnson, C.R., James, S.J., Manning-Courtney, P. (2015). Dietary supplementation in children with autism spectrum disorders: common, insufficient, and excessive. *J Acad Nutr Diet,* [Epub ahead of print].

27. Graf-Myles, J., Farmer, C., Thurm, A., Royster, C., Kahn, P., Soskey, L., Rothschild, L., Swedo, S. (2013). Dietary adequacy of children with autism compared with controls and the impact of restricted diet. *J Dev Behav Pediatr,* 34(7), 449-459. Retrieved from www.ncbi.nlm.nih.gov/pmc/articles/PMC3819433/pdf/nihms505909.pdf

28. Whiteley, P., Shattock, P., Knivsberg, A-M., Seim, A., Reichelt, K.L., Todd, L., Carr, K., Hooper, M. (2013). Gluten- and casein-free dietary intervention for autism spectrum conditions. *Frontiers in Human Neuroscience*, 6, 1-08. Retrieved from www.ncbi.nlm.nih.gov/pmc/articles/PMC3819433/pdf/nihms505909.pdf

29. Generation Rescue. (2015). *Corporate sponsors.* Retrieved from www.generationrescue.org/sponsorship/our-sponsors/

30. Imran, S., Hussiana, Z., Ghaaafoor, F., Nagra, S.A., Ziai, N.A. (2013). Comparative effi-

ciency of different methods of gluten extraction in indigenous varieties of wheat. *Archivos Latinoamericanos de Nutricion*, 63(2), 180-188.

31. Pusponegoro, H.D., Ismael, S., Firmansyah, A., Sastroasmoro, S., Vandenplas, Y. (2015). Gluten and casein supplementation does not increase symptoms in children with autism spectrum disorder. *Acta Paediatr.* [Epub ahead of print].

32. Buie, T. (2013). The relationship of autism and gluten. *Clin Ther*, 35(5), 578-583.

33. Mari-Bauset, S. Zazpe, I., Mari-Sanchis, A., Llopis-Gonzalez, A., Morales-Suarez-Varela, M. (2014). Evidence of the gluten-free and casein-free diet in autism spectrum disorders: a systematic review. *J Child Neurol*, 29(12), 1718-1727

34.Lacasana, M., Lopez-Flores, I., Rodriguez-Barranco, M., Aguilar-Garduno, C., Blanco-Munoz, J., Perez-Mendez, O., Gonzales-Alzaga, B., Bassol, S., Cebrian, M.E. (2010). Interaction between organophosphate pesticide exposure and PON1 activity on thyroid function. *Toxicol Appl Pharmacol*, 249(1), 16-24.

35. Detweiler, M.B. (2014). Organophosphate intermediate syndrome with neurological complications of extrapyramidla symptoms in clinical practice. *J Neurosci Rural Prac*, 5(3), 298-301. Retrieved from www.ncbi.nlm.nih.gov/pmc/articles/PMC4078626/

36. Kellman, R. (2011). The thyroid-autism connection: the role of endocrine disruptors. *Journal of Autism One*, 2, 111-117. Retrieved from http://nancymullanmd.com/pdf/TheThyroidAutismConnection.pdf

37. Catassi, C., Gatti, S., & Fasano, A. (2014). The new epidemiology of celiac disease. *Journal of Pediatric Gastroenterology & Nutrition*, 59:S7-S9. http://journals.lww.com/jpgn/Fulltext/2014/07001/The_New_Epidemiology_of_Celiac_Disease.5.aspx

38. Pamela's Products. (2015). *Donations, samples, event requests.* Retrieved from www.pamelasproducts.com/donation-request/

39. Delightfully Gluten Free. (2015). *Bob's birthday club for autism.* Retrieved from http://delightfullyglutenfree.com/2012/05/bobs-birthday-club-for-autism/

40. Ryckman, K. (2014). *Donation for "tee it up for autism" event.* Retrieved from http://betterbatter.org/?s=autism&submit.x=0&submit.y=0

41. Reid, I.R., Bristow, S.M., Bolland, M.J. (2015). Calcium supplements: benefits and risks. *J Intern Med*, [Epub ahead of print]. www.ncbi.nlm.nih.gov/pubmed/26174589

42. Stickel, F., Shouval, D. (2015). Hepatotoxicity of herbal and dietary supplements: an update. *Arch Toxicol*, 89(6), 851-865.

43. Genuis, S.J., Schwalfenberg, G., Siy, A-K., J., Rodushkin, I. (2012). Toxic element contamination of natural health products and pharmaceutical preparations. *PLOS ONE*, 7(11), e49676. Retrieved from www.ncbi.nlm.nih.gov/pmc/articles/PMC3504157/pdf/pone .0049676.pdf

44. Food and Drug Administration. (2015). *Are dietary supplements approved by the FDA?* Retrieved from www.fda.gov/AboutFDA/Transparency/Basics/ucm194344.htm

45. Food and Drug Administration. (2016). *Dietary supplements: what you need to know.* Retrieved from www.fda.gov/Food/ResourcesForYou/Consumers/ucm109760.htm

46. Food and Drug Administration. (2016). *How to report product problems and complaints to the FDA.* Retrieved from www.fda.gov/ForConsumers/ConsumerUpdates/ucm 049087.htm

CHAPTER 8

1. U.S. Department of Health and Human Services, U. S. Department of Agriculture. (2015). *2015-2020 dietary guidelines for Americans, 8th edition.* Retrieved from https://health.gov/dietaryguidelines/2015/guidelines/

2. The National Academies Press, Institute of Medicine. (2005). *Dietary reference intakes for energy, carbohydrate, fiber, fat, fatty acids, cholesterol, protein, and amino acids (macronutrients).* Retrieved from www.nap.edu/download/10490

3. European Food Information Council. (2015). *Facts on fats—dietary fats and health.* Retrieved from www.eufic.org/article/en/page/RARCHIVE/expid/Facts_on_Fats_Dietary_Fats_and_Health/

4. U.S. National Library of Medicine, (2017). *Facts about polyunsaturated fats.* Retrieved from https://medlineplus.gov/ency/patientinstructions/000747.htm

5. Abedin, L., Lien, E.L., Vingrys, A.J., & Sinclair, A.J. (1999). The effects of dietary alpha-linolenic acid compared with docosahexaenoic acid on brain, retina, liver, and heart in the guinea pig. *Lipids,* 34(5):475-482.

6. White, B. (2009). Dietary fatty acids. *American Family Physician,* 80(4):345-350. Retrieved from www.aafp.org/afp/2009/0815/p345.html

7. Reece, J.B., Taylor, M.R., Simon, E.J., Dickey, J.L., Hogan, K. (Ed.). (2015). *Campbell biology: concepts & connections.* Upper Saddle River, NJ: Pearson

8. Mozaffarian, D., et al. (2006). Trans fatty acids and cardiovascular disease. *New England Journal of Medicine,* 354:1601-1613.

9. National Cancer Institute. (2016). *Top food sources of saturated fat among the U.S. population, 2005-2006.* Retrieved from http://epi.grants.cancer.gov/diet/foodsources/sat_fat/sf.html

10. United States Food and Drug Administration. (2016). *Trans fats.* Retrieved from www.fda.gov/Food/ucm292278.htm

11. Dyall, S.C. (2015). Long-chain omega-3 fatty acids and the brain: a review of the independent and shared effects of EPA, DPA, and DHA. *Frontiers in Aging Neuroscience,* 7:52. Retrieved from www.ncbi.nlm.nih.gov/pmc/articles/PMC4404917/pdf/fnagi-07-00052.pdf

12. Parletta, N., Niyonsenga, T., & Duff, J. (2016). Omega-3 and omega-6 polyunsaturated fatty acid levels and correlations with symptoms in children with attention deficit hyperactivity disorder, autism spectrum disorder and typically developing controls. *PLoS ONE,* 11(5). Retrieved from www.ncbi.nlm.nih.gov/pmc/articles/PMC4883772/pdf/pone.0156432.pdf

13. Arterburn, L.M., Oken, H.A., Bailey, H.E., Hamersley, J., Kuratko, C.N., Hoffman, J.P. (2008). Algal-oil capsules and cooked salmon: nutritionally equivalent sources of docosahexaenoic acid. *J Am Diet Assoc,* 108(7), 1204-1209.

14. Food and Drug Administration. (2015). *What you need to know about mercury in fish and shellfish (brochure).* Retrieved from www.fda.gov/food/resourcesforyou/consumers/ucm110591.htm

15. Dufault, R., Lukiw, W.J., Crider, R., Schnoll, R., Wallinga, D., & Deth, R. (2012). A macroepigenetic approach to identify the factors responsible for the autism epidemic in the United States. *Clinical Epigenetics,* 4:6. Retrieved from www.clinicalepigeneticsjournal .com/content/4/1/6

16. Dufault, R., Schnoll, R., Lukiw, W.J., LeBlanc, B., Cornett, C., Patrick, L., Wallinga, D., Gilbert, S.G., & Crider, R. (2009). Mercury exposure, nutritional deficiencies and metabolic disruptions may affect learning in children. *Behavioral and Brain Functions,* 5:44. Retrieved from www.ncbi.nlm.nih.gov/pmc/articles/PMC2773803/#!po=76.0417

17. Dufault, R., Berg, Z., Crider, R., Schnoll R., Wetsit, L., Two Bulls, W., Gilbert, S., Kingston, S., Wolle, M., Rahman, M., & Laks, D. (2015). Blood inorganic mercury is directly associated with glucose levels in the human population and may be linked to processed food intake. *Integrative Molecular Medicine,* 2(3), 166-179. Retrieved from http://oatext.com/pdf/IMM-2-134.pdf

18. Emmett, P.M., Jones, L.R., & Golding, J. (2015). Pregnancy diet and associated outcomes in the Avon longitudinal study of parents and children. *Nutrition Reviews,* 73(S3):154-174. Retrieved from www.ncbi.nlm.nih.gov/pmc/articles/PMC4586451/pdf/ nuv053.pdf

19. Kuratko, C.N., Barrett, E.C., Nelson, E.B., Salem, N. (2013). The relationship of docosa-hexaenoic acid (DHA) with learning and behavior in healthy children: a review. *Nutrients,* 5, 2777-2810. Retrieved from www.ncbi.nlm.nih.gov/pmc/articles/PMC3738999/pdf/ nutrients-05-02777.pdf

20. van Elst, K., Bruining, H., Birtoli, B., Terreaux, C., Buitelaar, J.K., Kas, M.J. (2014). Food for thought: dietary changes in essential fatty acid ratios and the increase in autism spectrum disorders. *Neurosci Biobehav Rev,* 45, 369-378.

21. Bos, D.J., Oranje, B., Veerhoek, E.S., Van Diepen, R.M., Weusten, J.M., Demmelmair, H., Koletzko, B., de Sain-van der Velden, M.G., Eilander, A., Hoeksma, M., Durston, S. (2015). Reduced symptoms of inattention after dietary omega-3 fatty acid supplementation in boys with and without attention deficit/hyperactivity disorder. *Neuropsychopharmacology,* Epub ahead of print

22. United States Environmental Protection Agency. (1997). Mercury study report to congress. Retrieved from www.epa.gov/mercury/mercury-study-report-congress

23. United States Food and Drug Administration. (1995). *Mercury in fish: cause for concern?*Retrieved from www.fda.gov/OHRMS/DOCKETS/ac/02/briefing/3872_Advisory%207.pdf

24. Suphioglu, C., De Mel, D., Kumar, L., Sadli, N., Freestone, D., Michalczyk, A., Sinclair, A., Ackland, M.L. (2010). The omega-3 fatty acid, DHA, decreases neuronal cell death in association with zinc transport. *FEBS Lett,* 584(3), 612-618. Retrieved from www.sciencedi-rect.com/science/article/pii/S001457930901059X

25. Krishna, S.S., Majumdar, I., & Grishin, N.V. (2003). Structural classification of zinc fingers. *Nucleic Acids Research,* 31(2):532-550. Retrieved from http://nar.oxfordjournals.org/ content/31/2/532.full.pdf+html

26. Solomons, N.W. (2013). Update on zinc biology. *Anuuals Nutrition and Metabolism,* 62 Suppl, 1:8-17.

27. United States Department of Agriculture. (2016). *USDA food composition databases.* Retrieved from https://ndb.nal.usda.gov/ndb/search/list

28. United States Department of Agriculture, Agricultural Research Service. (2005). USDA national nutrient database for standard reference, release 18: foods high in zinc. Nutrient Data Laboratory.

29. Grimes, C.A., Szymlek-Gay, E.A., Campbell, K.J., & Nicklas, T.A. (2015). Food sources of total energy and nutrients among U.S. infants and toddlers: National Health and Nutrition Examination Survey 2005-2012. *Nutrients, 7,* 6797-6836. Retrieved from www.ncbi.nlm.nih.gov/pmc/articles/PMC4555149/

30. Pasiakos, S.M., Agarwal, S., Lieberman, H.R., & Fulgoni, V.L. (2015). Sources and amounts of animal, diary, and plant protein intake of U.S. adults in 2007-2010. *Nutrients, 7,* 7058-7069. Retrieved from www.ncbi.nlm.nih.gov/pmc/articles/PMC4555161/

31. Beasley, J.M., Deierlein, A.L., Morland, K.B., Granieri, E.C., & Spark, A. (2016). Is meeting the recommended dietary allowance (RDA) for protein related to body composition among older adults?: Results from the cardiovascular health of seniors and build environment study. *Journal of Nutrition and Healthy Aging,* 20(8):790-796.

32. Berryman, C.E., Agarwal, S., Lieberman, H.R., Fulgoini, V.L., & Pasiakos, S.M. (2016). Diets higher in animal and plant protein are associated with lower adiposity and do not impair kidney function in U.S. adults. *American Journal of Clinical Nutrition,* 104(3):743-749.

33. Lustig, R.H. (2013). Fructose: it's "alcohol without the buzz." *Advances in Nutrition,* 4(2):226-235. Retrieved from www.ncbi.nlm.nih.gov/pmc/articles/PMC3649103/

34. Bashiardes, S., Shapiro, H., Rozin, S., Shibolet, O., & Elinav, E. (2016). Non-alcoholic fatty liver and the gut microbiota. *Molecular Metabolism,* 5(9):782-784. Retrieved from www.ncbi.nlm.nih.gov/pmc/articles/PMC5004228/

35. Softic, S., Cohen, D.E., & Kahn, C.R. (2016). Role of dietary fructose and hepatic de novo lipogenesis in fatty liver disease. *Digestive Diseases & Sciences,* 61(5):1282-1293. Retrieved from http://link.springer.com/article/10.1007%2Fs10620-016-4054-0

36. Basaranoglu, M., Basaranoglu, G., Sabuncu, T., & Senturk, H. (2013). Fructose as a key player in the development of fatty liver disease. *World Journal of Gastroenterology,* 19(8):1166-1172. Retrieved from www.ncbi.nlm.nih.gov/pmc/articles/PMC3587472/

37. Jin, R., & Vos, M.B. (2015). Fructose and liver function—is this behind nonalcoholic liver disease? *Current Opinion Clinical Nutrition and Metabolic Care,* 18(5):490-495.

38. Jinjuvadia, R., Antaki, F., Lohia, P., & Liangpunsakul, S. (2016). The association between nonalcoholic fatty liver disease and metabolic abnormalities in the United States population. *Journal of Clinical Gastroenterology,* E-pub ahead of print.

39. Hamza, R.T., Ahmed, A.Y., Rezk, D.G., & Hamed, A.I. (2016). Dietary fructose intake in obese children and adolescents: relation to procollagen type III N-terminal peptide (P3NP) and non-alcoholic fatty liver disease. *Journal of Pediatric Endocrinology and Metabolism,* E-pub ahead of print.

40. Lustig, R.H., et al. (2016). Isocaloric fructose restriction and metabolic improvement in children with obesity and metabolic syndrome. *Obesity,* 24(2):453-460.

41. Younossi, Z.M. et al. (2016). The economic and clinical burden of nonalcoholic fatty liver disease in the United States and Europe. *Hepatology,* 64(5):1577-1586.

42. Case, A., & Deaton, A. (2015). Rising morbidity and mortality in midlife among white non-Hispanic Americans in the 21st century. *Proceedings of the National Academy of Sciences,* 112(49):15078-15083. Retrieved from www.ncbi.nlm.nih.gov/pmc/articles/PMC4679063/pdf/pnas.201518393.pdf

43. United States National Library of Medicine. (2016). *Carbohydrates.* Retrieved from https://medlineplus.gov/ency/article/002469.htm

44. Mozaffarian, D., Hao, T., Rimm, E.B., Willett, W.C., & Hu, F.B. (2011). Changes in diet and lifestyle and long-term weight gain in women and men. *New England Journal of Medicine,* 364:2392-2404. Retrieved from www.ncbi.nlm.nih.gov/pmc/articles/PMC3151731/

45. Merchant, A.T. et al. (2009). Carbohydrate intake and overweight and obesity among healthy adults. *Journal of the American Dietetic Association,* 109(7):1165-1172. Retrieved from www.ncbi.nlm.nih.gov/pmc/articles/PMC3093919/pdf/nihms285117.pdf

46. Lu, C., Barr, D.B., Pearson, M.A., & Waller, L.A. (2008). Dietary intake and its contribution to longitudinal organophosphorus pesticide exposure in urban/suburban children. *Environmental Health Perspectives,* 116(4):537-542. Retrieved from www.ncbi.nlm.nih.gov/pmc/articles/PMC2290988/

47. Curl, C.L., Fenske, R.A., & Elgethun, K. (2003). Organophosphorus pesticide exposure of urban and suburban preschool children with organic and conventional diets. *Environmental Health Perspectives,* 111(3):377-382. Retrieved from www.ncbi.nlm.nih.gov/pmc/articles/PMC1241395/

48. Bradman, A., et al. (2015). Effect of organic diet intervention on pesticide exposures in young children living in low-income urban and agricultural communities. *Environmental Health Perspectives,* 123(10):1086-1093. Retrieved from www.ncbi.nlm.nih.gov/pmc/articles/PMC4590750/

49. Krol, W.J., Arsenault, T.L., Pylypiw, H.M., & Mattina, M.J.I. (2000). Reduction of pesticide residues by rinsing. *Journal of Agriculture and Food Chemistry,* 48:4666-4670.

50. Krol, W.J., Arsenault, T.L., & Mattina, M.J.I. (2000). Pesticide residues in food sold in Connecticut 1999. *Connecticut Agricultural Experiment Station Bulletin,* 964, April.

51. National Pesticide Information Center. (2016). *Minimizing pesticide residues in food.* Retrieved from http://npic.orst.edu/health/foodprac.html

52. Halken, S. (2004). Prevention of allergic disease in childhood: clinical and epidemiological aspects of primary and secondary allergy prevention. *Pediatric Allergy and Immunology,* Suppl 16:4-5, 9-32.

53. Austin, D.W., Spolding, B., Gondalia, S., Shandley, K., Palombo, E.A., Knowles, S., Walder, K. (2014). Genetic variation associated with hypersensitivity to mercury. *Toxicol Int,* 21(3), 236-241. Retrieved from www.ncbi.nlm.nih.gov/pmc/articles/PMC4413404/

54. Petrus, N.C.M. et al. (2016). Cow's milk allergy in Dutch children: an epigenetic pilot study. *Clinical & Translational Allergy,* 6:16. Retrieved from www.ncbi.nlm.nih.gov/pmc/articles/PMC4855719/

55. Quake, C., & Nadeau, K.C. (2015). The role of epigenetic mediation and the future of food allergy research. *Semin Cell Dev Bio,* 43:125-130.

56. Furlong, C.E., et al. (2005). Role of paraoxonase (PON1) status in pesticide sensitivity: genetic and temporal determinants. *Neurotoxicology,* 26(4):651-659.

57. Rapp, D. J. (1996). *Is this your child's world?* New York, NY: Bantam Books.

58. Valenta, R., Hochwallner, H., Linhart, B., & Pahr, S. (2015). Food allergies: the basics. *Gastroenterology,* 148(6):1120-1131. Retrieved from www.ncbi.nlm.nih.gov/pmc/articles/PMC4414527/

59. Alabdali, A., Al-Ayadhi, L., & El-Ansary, A. (2014). A key role for an impaired detoxification mechanism in the etiology and severity of autism spectrum disorders. *Behavioral and Brain Functions,* 10:14. Retrieved from www.behavioralandbrainfunctions.com/content/10/1/14

60. Woo, H.D., Kim, D.W., Hong, Y-S., Kim, Y-M., Seo, J-H., Choe, B.M., Park, J.H., Kang, J-W., Yoo, J-H., Chueh, H.W., Lee, J.H., Kwak, M.J., & Kim, J. (2014). Dietary patterns in children with attention deficit/hyperactivity disorder (ADHD). *Nutrients,* 6, 1539-1553. Retrieved from www.ncbi.nlm.nih.gov/pmc/articles/PMC4011050/

CONCLUSION

1. U.S. Food and Drug Administration. (2016). *FSMA final rule for preventive controls for human food.* Retrieved from www.fda.gov/Food/GuidanceRegulation/FSMA/ucm334115.htm#Key_Requirements

2. U.S. Food and Drug Administration. (2016). *Standards for produce safety.* Retrieved from www.fda.gov/downloads/Food/GuidanceRegulation/FSMA/UCM472499.pdf

3. U.S. Food and Drug Administration. (2016). *FSMA final rule on produce safety.* Retrieved from www.fda.gov/Food/GuidanceRegulation/FSMA/ucm334114.htm

4. U.S. Food and Drug Administration. (2016). *President's fiscal year 2017 budget request: key investments for implementing the FDA food safety modernization act (FMSA).* Retrieved from www.fda.gov/Food/GuidanceRegulation/FSMA/ucm432576.htm

5. U.S. Centers for Disease Control and Prevention. (2016). *Estimates of foodborne illness.* Retrieved from www.cdc.gov/foodborneburden/index.html

6. Scallan, E. et al. (2011). Foodborne illness acquired in the United States—major pathogens. *Emerging Infectious Diseases,* 17(1):7-15. Retrieved from wwwnc.cdc.gov/eid/article/17/1/pdfs/p1-1101.pdf

7. Kochanek, K.D., Murphy, S.L., Xu, J., & Tejada-Vera, B. (2016). Deaths: final data for 2014. *National Vital Statistics Reports,* 65(4):1-122. Retrieved from www.cdc.gov/nchs/data/nvsr/nvsr65/nvsr65_04.pdf

8. U.S. Food and Drug Administration. (2016). *FDA cuts trans fat in processed foods.* Retrieved from www.fda.gov/ForConsumers/ConsumerUpdates/ucm372915.htm

9. Schutze, I., & Muller, W. (1979). Determination of trace elements in dietary fats and emulsifiers by non-flame atomic absorption spectrometry (AAS). 2. Determination of mercury in dietary fats and emulsifiers. *Nahrung,* 23(9-10):867-874.

10. Azevedo, B.F., et al. (2012). Toxic effects of mercury on the cardiovascular and central nervous systems. *Journal of Biomedicine and Biotechnology,* 1-11. Retrieved from www.hindawi.com/journals/bmri/2012/949048/

11. Dufault, R., Berg, Z., Crider, R., Schnoll R., Wetsit, L., Two Bulls, W., Gilbert, S., Kingston, S., Wolle, M., Rahman, M., & Laks, D. (2015). Blood inorganic mercury is directly associated with glucose levels in the human population and may be linked to

processed food intake. *Integrative Molecular Medicine,* 2(3), 166-179. Retrieved from http://oatext.com/pdf/IMM-2-134.pdf

12. Centers for Disease Control and Prevention (CDC). (2013). *National health education standards.* Retrieved from www.cdc.gov/healthyschools/sher/standards/index.htm

13. Centers for Disease Control and Prevention (CDC). (2013). *Guideline 5.* Retrieved from www.cdc.gov/healthyschools/npao/healthed.htm

14. Lenders, C., et al. (2013). A novel nutrition medicine education model: The Boston University experience. *Advances in Nutrition,* 4(1), 1-7.

15. Sylvetsky, A. C., et al. (2013). Youth understanding of healthy eating and obesity: A focus group study. *Journal of Obesity.* doi:10.1155/2013/670295

16. Miller, L. M. S., Gibson, T. N., & Applegate, E. A. (2010). Predictors of nutrition information comprehension in adulthood. *Patient Education and Counseling, 80*(1), 107-112.

17. Lopaczynski, W. (2012). Translational research and behavioral sciences in developmental medicine: Metabolic conditions of pregnancy versus autism spectrum disorders. *Medycyna Wieku Rozwojowego, 16*(3), 171-174. Retrieved from http://medwiekurozwoj.pl/articles/2012-3-1.pdf

18. Dufault, R., Lukiw, W. J., Crider, R., Schnoll, R., Wallinga, D., & Deth, R. (2012). A macro epigenetic approach to identify factors responsible for the autism epidemic in the United States. *Clinical Epigenetics, 4,* 6. Retrieved from www.ncbi.nlm.nih.gov/pmc/articles/PMC3378453/pdf/1868-7083-4-6.pdf

19. Sullivan, E. L., Smith, M. S., & Grove, K. L. (2011). Perinatal exposure to high-fat diet programs energy balance, metabolism and behavior in adulthood. *Neuroendocrinology, 93*(1), 1-8. Retrieved from www.ncbi.nlm.nih.gov/pmc/articles/PMC3700139/pdf/nen-0093-0001.pdf

20. U.S. Department of Agriculture (USDA). (2013). *Women, infants, and children (WIC).* Retrieved from www.fns.usda.gov/wic/women-infants-and-children-wic

21. Shamberger, R. J. (2011). Autism rates associated with nutrition and the WIC program. *Journal of the American College of Nutrition, 30*(5), 348-353.

22. Durkin, M. S., et al. (2010). Socioeconomic inequality in the prevalence of autism spectrum disorder: Evidence from a U.S. cross-sectional study. *PLoS One, 5*(7), e11551. Retrieved from www.ncbi.nlm.nih.gov/pmc/articles/PMC2902521/pdf/pone.0011551.pdf

23. Thomas, P., Zahorodny, W., Peng, B., Kim, S., Jani, N., Halperin, W., & Brimacombe, M. (2012). The association of autism diagnosis with socioeconomic status. *Autism, 16*(2), 201-213.

24. Food Ingredient and Health Research Institute. (2017). *Safe and Healthy Diet Tutor.* Retrieved from www.foodingredient.info/safehealthydiettutor.html

25. Food Ingredient and Health Research Institute. (2017). *Syllabus.* Retrieved from www.foodingredient.info/safehealthydiettutor/syllabus.html

RESOURCES

1. Food Ingredient and Health Research Institute. (2017). *Syllabus.* Retrieved from www.foodingredient.info/safehealthydiettutor/syllabus.html

About the Author

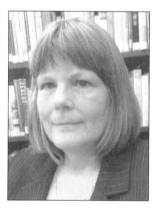

Renee Dufault, BS, MAT, DHEd, joined the Army after graduating high school to become a medical laboratory specialist and earn the GI bill. After her four-year stint in the Army, she earned her undergraduate degree in environmental policy analysis and planning at the University of California at Davis. She served in the Navy for two years as an Industrial Hygiene Officer. She then transferred to the Public Health Service (PHS), where she served as an Environmental Health Officer. During her fourteen-year PHS career, she worked at the National Institutes of Health, Environmental Protection Agency (EPA), Shoshone-Paiute Tribes, and the Food and Drug Administration (FDA), where she provided expertise in the areas of toxicology, environmental health, and industrial hygiene.

After twenty years with the uniformed service, she retired early to publish her findings of mercury in high fructose corn syrup and continue her research with collaborators on the role toxic food ingredients play in the development of disease conditions. Her most popular article to date was published in the *Clinical Epigenetics* journal (Dufault et al., 2012) and explores the gene-environment interactions responsible for the autism epidemic in the United States. The article has been downloaded over 150,000 times and continues to be highly cited by other scientists.

Since her early retirement, Renee completed her doctorate degree in Health Education and has quietly collaborated with scientists worldwide to conduct studies and publish articles in medical journals that explain how toxic substances enter the food supply, endangering child health and development. Dr. Dufault is the founding Executive Director of the Food Ingredient and Health Research Institute (FIHRI). She is an invited guest speaker at conferences throughout the world. She was a distinguished keynote speaker at the Clinical Epigenetics Society meeting in Germany and the Learning Disabilities Association of America conference in San Antonio, Texas. Dr. Dufault was invited by the Smithsonian Institute to present the results of a clinical trial conducted to determine the role dietary inorganic mercury plays in the development of type 2 diabetes among American Indians. A video of the presentation was shared by the National Museum of the American Indian on YouTube and remains freely available to the public. She spoke at the Neurological Disorders Summit in San Francisco, California, where she gave a lecture on prenatal nutrition from an epigenetic perspective to optimize birth outcomes.

While Dr. Dufault's busy schedule takes her around the world, she resides in Hawai'i. In her spare time, Dr. Dufault visits with her two grown children and their families in California and New York. She has four grandchildren who bring her much joy.

Index

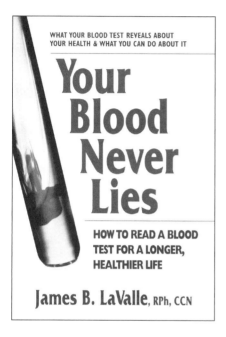

WHAT YOUR BLOOD TEST REVEALS ABOUT
YOUR HEALTH & WHAT YOU CAN DO ABOUT IT

Your Blood Never Lies

HOW TO READ A BLOOD
TEST FOR A LONGER,
HEALTHIER LIFE

James B. LaValle, RPh, CCN

YOUR BLOOD NEVER LIES

How to Read a Blood Test
for a Longer, Healthier Life

James B. LaValle, RPh, CCN

If you're like most people, you probably rely on your doctor to interpret the results of your blood tests, which contain a wealth of information on the state of your health. A blood test can tell you how well your kidneys and liver are functioning, your potential for heart disease and diabetes, the strength of your immune system, the chemical profile of your blood, and many other important facts about the state of your health. And yet, most of us cannot decipher these results ourselves, nor can we even formulate the right questions to ask about them—or we couldn't, until now.

In *Your Blood Never Lies,* best-selling author Dr. James LaValle clears the mystery surrounding blood test results. In simple language, he explains all the information found on a typical lab report—the medical terminology, the numbers and percentages, and the laboratory jargon—and makes it accessible. This means that you will be able to look at your own blood test results and understand the significance of each biological marker being measured. To help you take charge of your health, Dr. LaValle also recommends the most effective standard and complementary treatments for dealing with any problematic findings. Rounding out the book are explanations of lab values that do not appear on the standard blood test, but that should be requested for a more complete picture of your current physiological condition.

A blood test can reveal so much about your body, but only if you can interpret the results. *Your Blood Never Lies* provides the up-to-date information you need to understand your results and take control of your life.

$16.95 • 368 pages • 6 x 9-inch paperback • ISBN 978-0-7570-0350-9

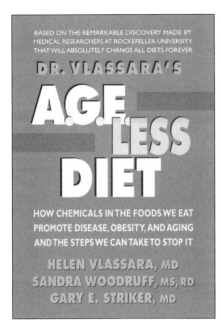

DR. VLASSARA'S A.G.E.-LESS DIET

How Chemicals in the Foods We Eat Promote Disease, Obesity, and Aging And the Steps We Can Take to Stop It

Helen Vlassara, MD, Sandra Woodruff, MS, RD, and Gary E. Striker, MD

Imagine naturally occurring toxins that are directly responsible for inflammation, chronic diseases, and aging. While that may not have been what Dr. Helen Vlassara was looking for when she began her work at the research laboratories of Rockefeller University, it was what her pioneering team discovered in 1985. Trying to understand why patients with diabetes were prone to develop heart, eye, kidney, nerve, and circulatory disorders, as well as other signs of premature aging, the team focused on compounds called *advanced glycation end products,* or *AGEs.*

Dr. Vlassara's research revealed that AGEs enter the body through the digestive tract via the diet, and that there is a tremendous difference between an AGE-laden diet and an AGE-less diet. AGEs simply accelerate the body's aging process by increasing oxidation and free radicals, hardening tissue, and creating chronic inflammation.

For years, these amazing studies have remained relatively unknown to the public and even the medical community. Now, Dr. Helen Vlassara and best-selling author Sandra Woodruff have written a complete guide to understanding what AGEs are and how you can avoid them through the careful selection of foods and cooking techniques. In *Dr. Vlassara's AGE-less Diet,* the authors offer simple principles that can be applied to your diet—or to any popular diet— to lower your intake of AGEs. They include an AGE ranking of foods as well as recipes that reduce your consumption of AGEs.

By lowering your AGE levels, you can reduce the potential of developing any number of serious disorders, look years younger, and enjoy greater health and longevity. *Dr. Vlassara's AGE-less Diet* guides you in making a real and important difference in your life.

$16.95 • 328 pages • 6 x 9-inch paperback • ISBN 978-0-7570-0420-9

SUICIDE BY SUGAR

A Startling Look at Our #1 National Addiction

Nancy Appleton, PhD, and G.N. Jacobs

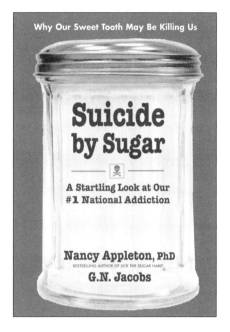

It is a dangerous, addictive white powder that can be found in abundance throughout this country. It is not illegal. In fact, it is available in or near playgrounds, schools, workplaces, homes, and vacation spots. It is in practically everything we eat and drink, and, once we're hooked on it, the cravings can be overwhelming. This white substance of abuse is sugar. Once associated only with cavities and simple weight gain, it is now linked to a host of devastating health conditions including cancer, epilepsy, dementia, hypoglycemia, obesity, and more. In this book, sugar addiction expert Dr. Nancy Appleton and health writer G.N. Jacobs not only expose the exorbitant levels of sugar we ingest, but also document the connection between our current health crisis and our sweet tooth.

Suicide by Sugar begins with the story of Dr. Appleton's battle with her own sugar addiction. Next, the authors examine all the frightening (and unknown) things that can go wrong when people consume too much sugar—from increased susceptibility to disease to imbalanced body chemistry. They go on to discuss the various ways scientists measure sugar's impact on blood glucose, and explain why these statistics cannot be solely relied on when choosing foods. The authors provide shocking information about the amount of sugar found in many popular foods and beverages, and an in-depth discussion of the ailments now associated with excessive sugar consumption. Finally, Dr. Appleton's easy-to-follow, effective lifestyle plan—complete with recipes—guides you in eliminating sugar from your life.

As children, we fall under the spell of ads that lure us to indulge in all things sweet. Is it any wonder that as adults, so few of us can see the dark side of sugar? *Suicide by Sugar* shines a bright light on our nation's addiction and helps us begin the journey toward health.

$15.95 • 192 pages • 6 x 9-inch paperback • ISBN 978-0-7570-0306-6

KILLER COLAS

The Hard Truth About Soft Drinks

Nancy Appleton, PhD, and G.N. Jacobs

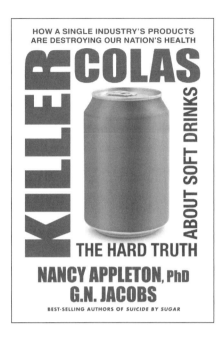

It's as American as fast food, ice cream, and apple pie. So why are people saying all those nasty things about soda? The answer is simple: Those nasty things are all true. While the facts may be hard to swallow, it is high time we address the damage being done to our well-being due to our long-running love affair with soft drinks and other sweetened beverages. In *Killer Colas,* Dr. Nancy Appleton and G.N. Jacobs provide a startling picture of an industry hell-bent on making a hefty profit at the ultimate expense of the country's health.

Over the last few decades, the sale of soft drinks, energy beverages, sports drinks, and enhanced waters has exploded, as has the incidence of obesity, diabetes, hypertension, heart disease, cancer, and stroke. *Killer Colas* looks at the origin of this downward spiral. The book traces the history and staggering growth of the soft drink industry, explores the powerful influence it has achieved through media-savvy advertising and marketing techniques, and examines the many harmful ingredients that these companies include in their most prized and popular formulas. In addition, it offers evidence of the frighteningly addictive properties of soft drinks, as well as research that links America's consumption of sweetened beverages to its overall decline in health.

In light of the country's overwhelming health crisis, the consequences of drinking soda and other sweetened beverages can no longer be ignored. *Killer Colas* exposes the facts behind a habit that is just as dangerous and destructive as smoking. Moreover, it suggests concrete solutions to this widespread problem, giving hope to a nation desperately in need of a healthful way forward. Once you have read this book, you will never look at soft drinks in the same way again.

$15.95 • 144 pages • 6 x 9-inch paperback • ISBN 978-0-7570-0341-7

HEALTH AT GUNPOINT

The FDA's Silent War Against Health Freedom

James J. Gormley

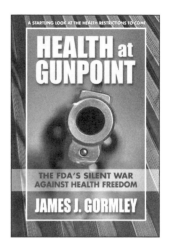

While the original intent of the Food and Drug Administration may have been honorable, over time, the mission has become tainted by lobbyists. *Health at Gunpoint* presents a history of the agency's long battle against health products and examines some of its most controversial decisions.

Now, the FDA is again poised to make decisions that would have a major impact on the public, this time, by imposing restrictions that could eliminate many of the nutritional supplements we take. *Health at Gunpoint* not only sheds light on what is happening, but also prepares us for the coming battle.

$14.95 • 176 pages • 6 x 9-inch paperback • ISBN 978-0-7570-0381-3

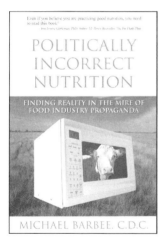

POLITICALLY INCORRECT NUTRITION

Finding Reality in the Mire of Food Industry Propaganda

Michael Barbee, CDC

Did you know that some artificial sweeteners can actually make you fat, or that certain soy products can upset your hormonal balance? *Politically Incorrect Nutrition* exposes many current beliefs foisted on both consumers and health-care practitioners by food industry propaganda. It analyzes popular claims and reveals what, in fact, is healthy—and what is decidedly *unhealthy*—by exploring objective scientific data on good nutrition.

If you want to provide the best possible food for yourself and your family, or if you simply want to learn the truth behind food myths, *Politically Incorrect Nutrition* is must reading.

$13.95 • 176 pages • 6 x 9-inch paperback • ISBN 978-1-890612-34-4

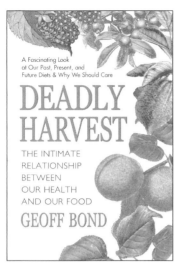

Deadly Harvest

The Intimate Relationship Between Our Health & Our Food

Geoff Bond

Contrary to what many people believe, the disorders that plague our society are not inevitable. Rather, they are the unfortunate result of modern dietary choices.

Using the latest scientific research and studies of primitive life, the author first explains the diet that our ancestors followed—one in harmony with the human species. He then describes how our present food choices affect our health, leading to disorders such as cancer, diabetes, and heart disease. Most important, he details measures we can take to improve both our diet and our quality of life.

$16.95 • 336 pages • 6 x 9-inch paperback • ISBN 978-0-7570-0142-0

GMO Free

Exposing the Hazards of Biotechnology to Ensure the Integrity of Our Food Supply

Mae-Wan Ho, PhD, and Lim Li Ching

The genetic engineering of crops constitutes a health crisis, yet the decision to use genetically modified organisms (GMOs) is currently being made for you by the government and multinational corporations. To combat this practice, over 600 scientists have called for a moratorium on the release of GMOs.

GMO Free takes a good look at the evidence scientists have compiled, and makes a strong case for a worldwide ban on GMO crops, to make way for sustainable agriculture and organic farming. It's time to take the future of your food supply into your own informed hands.

$10.95 • 152 pages • 5.5 x 8.5-inch paperback • ISBN 978-1-890612-37-5

**For more information about our books,
visit our website at www.squareonepublishers.com**